PHYSICIANS AND THE PEACE MOVEMENT

PHYSICIANS AND THE PEACE MOVEMENT
Prescriptions for Hope

NICK LEWER

Department of Peace Studies
University of Bradford

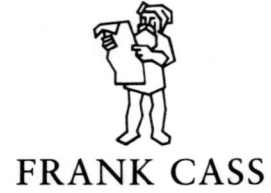

FRANK CASS

JX
1952
.L537
1992

First published in 1992 in Great Britain by
FRANK CASS & CO. LTD.
Gainsborough House, Gainsborough Road,
London E11 1RS, England

and in the United States of America by
FRANK CASS
c/o International Specialized Book Services, Inc.
5602 N.E. Hassalo Street, Portland, Oregon 97213

Copyright © 1992 Frank Cass & Co. Ltd.

British Library Cataloguing in Publication Data

Lewer, Nick
 Physicians and the peace movement : prescriptions
 for hope.
 I. Title
 372.172

ISBN 0-7146-3438-7

Library of Congress Cataloging-in-Publication Data

Lewer, Nick.
 Physicians and the peace movement : prescriptions for hope / Nick
Lewer.
   p.   cm.
 Includes bibliographical references and index.
 ISBN 0-7146-3438-7
 1. Peace movements. 2. Physicians. I. Title.
JX1952.L537   1992
  327.1'72'08861——dc20   91-16473
                                                      CIP

All rights reserved. No part of this publication may be reproduced in
any form or by any means, electronic, mechanical, photocopying,
recording or otherwise, without the prior permission of Frank Cass and
Company Limited.

Printed in Great Britain by BPCC Wheatons Ltd, Exeter

CONTENTS

INTRODUCTION 1

PART ONE

Conceptions of Peace 3
The Peace Movement and Approaches to Peace 5
Peaks and Troughs in the Peace Movement 7
Peace Studies and Peace Research 9
Physicians, War and Peace 10
   The Red Cross 11
   Social, Political and Ethical Responsibilities 11
Conclusion 15

PART TWO: 1815–1918

Pioneer Citizen Diplomats 16
   Benjamin Rush 16
   George Logan and Mediation 19
The First Peace Societies: 1815–43 20
Dr Rudolph Virchow 23
Dr Adolph Fischoff 25
Socialist and Feminist Influences 26
   Anna Kuliscioff 26
   Madeleine Pelletier 28
Albert Skarvan's Act of Individual Defiance 29
International Medical Association against War (IMAW) 30
Charles Richet and Idiot Man 32
Other Physician Pacifists Active before the First World War 33
The First World War (1914–18) 35
Fellowship of Reconciliation 36
Women Mobilise Against the War 37
Medical Thinking on the Causes of War 39

Dr Georg Friedrich Nicolai (1874–1964): The Tribal Instinct 39
Dr Wilfred Trotter (1872–1939): The Herd Instinct 41
Dr Sigmund Freud (1856–1939): The Primitive Instincts 42
November 1918: War Ends 44

PART THREE: 1919–45

Rise of Fascism 45
League of Nations 47
The 'Triple Crisis' of 1936 48
The Peace Movement after the First World War 48
   Women's International League for Peace and Freedom 48
   War Resisters International 49
   European Medical Peace Groups in the 1930s 50
Medical Peace Campaign: Great Britain 52
   The White Sickness 57
   Advice to Doctors from Dick Sheppard 57
Dr Maria Montessori: Educator for Peace 58
Role of the Red Cross Questioned 60
The Second World War (1939–45) 61

PART FOUR: 1946–90

Periods of Activity in the Peace Movement: A Summary 63
Medical Association for the Prevention of War 64
Doctors Confront Government War Planning 67
MAPW and the Labour Party: Proscription 68
MAPW and Professor Lionel Penrose 69
Doctors Protest about the H-bomb 70
Dr Albert Schweitzer: Nobel Peace Prize 1953 71
Pugwash 72
Sane 73
Increasing Nuclear Tensions 73
Physicians for Social Responsibility 74
Decline in Anti-nuclear Activity by the Peace Movement 76
MAPW in the 1960s and 1970s 77
Re-activation of the Peace Movement to Nuclear Issues 78
International Physicians for the Prevention of Nuclear War 78
Medical Campaign against Nuclear Weapons (UK) 80

British Medical Association and its Relations with MAPW and MCANW	82
The BMA and the Political Implications of the 1983 Report	83
Civil Defence Plans: Reaction from the Medical Peace Movement	85
The Role of Community Physicians	85
Faculty of Community Medicine	87
Disagreement over Casualty Calculations	88
Ethical Questions for Doctors in Considering Nuclear War	89
Contributions from Psychiatry and Psychology to the Nuclear Debate and Promotion of Peace	91
Defence Mechanisms: Why We Accept the Bomb	92
A Critique of Psychological Approaches to Peace and War Considerations	94
Clinical Approach	95
Social–Psychological Approach	95
Mediation and Conflict Resolution: Developing a New Role for Physicians and other Health Workers in Peacemaking Processes	96
CONCLUSION	99
NOTES	108
BIBLIOGRAPHY	123
INDEX	130

For Ailsa:
Thank you

INTRODUCTION

> There are subjects such as peace that our civilisation cannot afford *not* to study. In the issue of peace what is at stake in our times at certain levels is the intellectual, moral, and physical well being of individuals and groups. What is at stake at a global level is not only such well being but human survival.[1]

This book was written in recognition of the many physicians and other health workers who, since the formation of the first peace societies in 1815, have dedicated their lives in an attempt to make the world a more peaceful and just place to live. My own active participation began when I joined the Medical Association for the Prevention of War (MAPW). The aims of this organisation, formed in 1951, include: to consider the doctor's ethical responsibility in relation to war; to study the causes and consequences of war, including the environmental dimension; and to examine the psychological mechanisms by which people are conditioned to view war as a necessity. MAPW continues, as will be seen, a long tradition of involvement by physicians and other health workers in the issues of war and peace, justice, human rights and development – the concerns of which are inevitably interconnected.

This study identifies and acknowledges some of the individuals and organisations who have contributed directly to this peace work – any particular emphases are purely a personal choice. In compiling this book (from many sources) I was acutely aware of the constraints imposed by space and, in such a broad survey, there are inevitably gaps. The intention is to introduce the field in an attempt to illustrate the main issues and avenues that have motivated individuals and groups to work directly for peace. No attempt is made to delve in any great depth into the history of the peace movement as a whole, and reference is made to the more comprehensive texts available on the subject.

For decades schoolchildren have, on the whole, been taught to respect and emulate traditionally viewed heroic role-models: for example the famous warriors and pugnacious politicians who operated from positions of power and strength. The men and women in this book represent, for me, the real heroes and heroines. Their often lonely stands for peace and justice required, in many instances, the utmost strength and bravery. We should teach our children more about such people.

The book is organised in four parts. Part One starts with a consideration of some aspects of peace terminology — its concepts, approaches and periods of activity. A distinction is then made between peace research and peace studies, and finally mention is made of the Red Cross — the first truly international humanitarian medical and relief organisation to be formed, which impartially aided the victims of violent conflict.

The remaining three parts have been divided into historical periods: Part Two: 1815–1918: from the formation of the first peace societies to the end of the First World War; Part Three: 1919–45: from the end of the First World War to the end of the Second; Part Four: 1946–90: the Nuclear Age.

The Conclusion draws the threads together and considers some ways in which the health professions may contribute to peace work in the future.

I would like to thank Dr Peter van den Dungen of the Department of Peace Studies, University of Bradford, for his help and encouragement.

Nick Lewer
Bradford, 1990

PART ONE

CONCEPTIONS OF PEACE

The concept of peace varies between different people and groups depending on their secular, political or religious standpoints. This will be reflected in the thinking and actions of the physician peace workers, and their organisations, illustrated in the following chapters.

Peace, for many, is more than just the absence of war or other manifestations of strife – it is intimately linked with the ideas of justice and freedom. Adam Curle states:

> There are conditions of social injustice, economic exploitation and political oppression which, while they are not war itself, are by no means peaceful and often lead to war. This 'structural violence' is built into social structures and deprives its victims of jobs, food, health, education, political liberties and human dignity.[1]

James O'Connell says the idea of peace contains two basic elements: willing co-operation among persons for social and personal goals and the absence of violence (in the shape of direct physical, psychological or moral violence).[2] O'Connell's understanding of peace comes from St Augustine's definition – 'the tranquillity of order' – and he writes of peace:

> Positively, peace requires co-operation among persons and groups for aims that include security, justice and freedom; and, negatively, it seeks to eliminate force and violence. Each aim is important: security guarantees survival; justice provides the links of co-operation as well as the minimal equality without which peace remains fragile; and freedom, finally, gives worth to people who without freedom remain diminished. Yet if peace is a basic human aim, peace is a process within which it is accomplished.[3]

Traditionally, according to Chatfield, the concept of peace has had three components:[4]

a. A sense of juridicial order associated with the Latin word *pax*. Pax was the Roman Goddess of Peace, and the Roman concept of peace was linked with the concepts of law, order and mutual duty.
b. A sense of ethical social relationships conveyed by the Greek word *eirene* (after the Greek Goddess of Peace).
c. A sense of well-being that flows from spiritual wholeness, conveyed by the Hebrew, *shalom*.

Two other components are added by G. K. Wilson:[5] from the Sanskrit source the term *satyagrahavarda*, and from the Roman Catholic Church the word *pacis*. Satyagrahavarda is the study of spiritual, mental and corporal forces making for harmony in the individual and in society – the search for the motivating forces in peace and stability. In its doctrine of 'just war' the Roman Catholic church has introduced value elements into the conditions of peace.[6]

For Michael Banks[7] the term 'peace' consists of four components:

1. Peace as harmony: a utopian idea from which conflict has been banished.
2. Peace as order: with stability, life is seen to be made predictable and relatively safe by a minimum of political order.
3. Peace as justice: issues to consider include poverty (social injustice), ethnic oppression, political weakness (latent and manifest), human rights, punishment (for current and past offences).
4. Peace as conflict management: peace is not a state of general tranquillity, but rather a network of relationships full of energy and conflict, which are kept under societal control.

Peace processes do not aim at eliminating all conflict, just the destructive and violent elements of it. Conflict is both inevitable and necessary because people have basic human needs expressed in society through competing values and clashing interests. What is needed are methods of conflict management and conflict resolution that utilise non-violent means. For this to happen effectively on an international scale, nation states must eventually accept the requirement of renouncing the right to wage war in settling grievances, and promote, actively, alternative dispute resolution mechanisms.

These various aspects and concepts of peace will be reflected in the peace work of physicians and their organisations, as we will see later on.

THE PEACE MOVEMENT AND APPROACHES TO PEACE

The organised peace movement began simultaneously in the United States and Great Britain with the formation of the first peace societies in 1815, at the end of the Napoleonic Wars.[8] Michael Howard defines the early peace movement as '. . .the political organisation of middle-class liberals on a transnational basis to secure by education, agitation and propaganda, the abolition of war'.[9]

The peace movement today consists of a large number of groups and organisations with different ideological orientations and value motivations, working through varied activities and methods, in a loose coalition who 'seek to influence the attitudes of the public, and the decisions of government, the latter's decisions especially in foreign and military policies'.[10]

Bob Overy distinguishes three kinds of peace movement:[11] movements to eliminate all war (such as the Quakers, Peace Pledge Union, Fellowship of Reconciliation); movements to end or prevent a particular war (anti-Vietnam War organisations); and movements to prevent particular aspects of war (Campaign for Nuclear Disarmament, Campaign Against the Arms Trade, anti-Trident). Overy makes the distinction between the peace movement itself, which is anti-war, and its *concerns* – which are much wider. Today's peace movement activists tend to be involved with broader social and political concerns such as environmental issues, civil liberties, human rights and health and social welfare. Peace is not seen by them in isolation as an abstract idea, but as part of a more 'wholistic' view of the way life should be lived.

Nigel Young expands on Overy's categories of the peace movement and identifies nine groups of goals/objectives:

Goals and objectives in the peace movement[12]

Opposition to specific weapons or weapon types	Anti-nuclear, poison gas.
Opposition to weapon or foreign bases	Polaris, Trident, Cruise, US bases.

Opposition to arms races	Pre-1914, the 1930s, the 1960s, the 1980s.
Opposition to war as such	Pacifist, socialist anti-militarist, liberal, 'abolition of war through international law and arbitration'.
Opposition to types of war	Nuclear, aggressive, 'imperialist'.
Opposition to military service	Religious (conscientious objectors), socialist (capitalist wars), civil libertarian (liberal).
Opposition to specific wars	Boer, Algerian, Spanish, Vietnam, Falklands/Malvinas, etc.
Support for transformation of militaristic structures	Socialist, anarchist, Gandhian movements, revolutionary and alternativist (Utopian).
Non-violent social change	Positive, programmatic peace scenarios.

Physicians and other health workers have been active within these various groups, as will be demonstrated in the following pages.

Mention must be made, at this stage, of organisations and groups who believe that peace is best preserved through maintaining military strength, particularly the nuclear deterrent. These 'peace through strength' groups (such as the Coalition for Peace Through Security and the Committee for Peace through Freedom in the UK; and the Heritage Foundation and the Committee on the Present Danger in the US) operate on the right of the political spectrum.[13] Their philosophy for peace is more in sympathy with that of Vegetius (fourth century): 'Let him who desires peace, prepare for war'. These groups have actively campaigned against the anti-nuclear organisations specifically, more often than not with their own governments' implicit support. I have arbitrarily excluded these organisations from the 'peace movement' on ideological grounds.

PEAKS AND TROUGHS IN THE PEACE MOVEMENT

The history of the international peace movement shows periods of surges in activity (peaks) followed by periods of decline and apparent apathy (troughs). This wave pattern can be considered to consist of two different components which Philip Everts identifies as *prophetic minorities* and *coalition movements*.[14] The former group represents the historic continuity between the peaks, which occur at irregular intervals, and expresses generally radical goals of opposing all war and changing societal structure. The troughs and peaks, Everts postulates, are caused by the presence or absence of the coalition movements. The peaks usually occur when organisations and forms of organisation develop whose general concerns cystallise around specific issues and focus on specific societal or political goals. The coalitions do not aim at the total transformation of society, but at more concrete goals: to stop one particular war, or the abolition of a particular weapon or weapons system. Nigel Young supports this view and demonstrates the way in which the various *traditions* relate to the periodic waves of activism. He lists some examples and organisations of peace traditions and relates the strength of these traditions to the activity of the mass peace movements in Britain between 1815 and 1981 (see Figure 1).

The peace traditions: some examples/organisations[15]

1. Religious peace traditions	Religious pacifism, Society of Friends (Quakers), Pax Christi, International Fellowship of Reconciliation.
2. Liberal internationalism	League of Nations Association, National Peace Council, Union of Democratic Control, disarmament campaigns.
3. Anti-conscriptionism	(Single issue lobbies), WRI, PPU, NCCL, No Conscription Fellowship.
4. Socialist war resistance	WRI, END.
5. Socialist internationalism	Second international, END.

FIGURE 1
THE MASS PEACE MOVEMENTS IN BRITAIN, 1815–1981

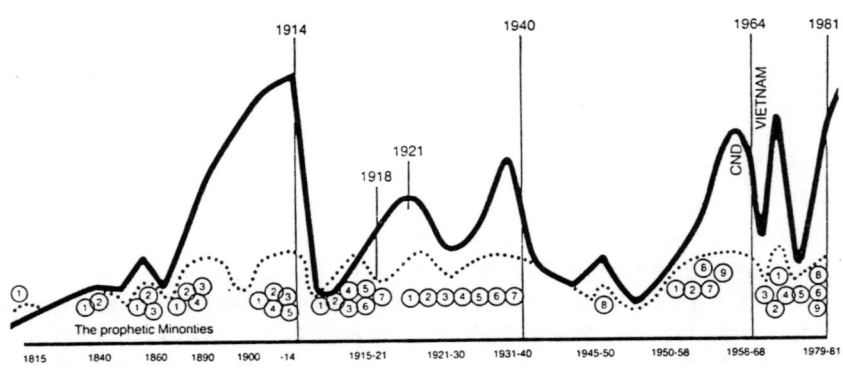

Notes: The numbers refer to the peace traditions. The dotted line suggests their strength as a whole in the given periods.

Source: Young, N. 'Tradition and innovation in the British Peace Movement: towards an analytical framework', in Taylor, R. and Young, N. (eds.), *Campaigns for Peace* (Manchester: University Press, 1987), p. 11. Reproduced with permission.

6. Feminist anti-militarism	WILPF, WFLOE, WONT.
7. Radical (secular) pacifism	Gandhian groups (Direct Action Committee), WRI, No More War Movement.
8. 'Comminternationalism'	Branches of the World Peace Council; peace committees.
9. Nuclear disarmament	CND, END, Committee of 100.
10. The 'new peace movement'	New Left, The Greens, END, 'Greenham Women'.

These traditions, and the role of physicians in them, both as individuals and as members of organisations, will be looked at in a historical context in the main text.

PEACE STUDIES AND PEACE RESEARCH

Peace studies and peace research are also known as peace science, conflict studies, world studies, conflict science and peace education. Since the late 1950s scholars have been actively engaged in an interdisciplinary approach to investigating the causes of conflict, violence and war and the problems of maintaining a condition of peace and of preventing war.[16] The new peace research methodology was heavily influenced by social sciences such as political science, sociology, social psychology, economics and rational choice theory. These subjects took precedence over the older traditionalist disciplines of diplomatic history, international law, and classical strategy. Advances in computer technology made it easier for social scientists to process large amounts of data and to run complex simulations of conflict. Mack[17] conceives of peace research as a collection of attributes which cluster together. It is characterised generally by a commitment to certain values and to policy-oriented research intended to realise those values: by a preference for the methods of the social sciences; by an enthusiasm for interdisciplinary research; by a conception of human nature which is more optimistic than that of the International Relations school of 'realists'; and by conceptions of 'peace' and 'violence' which are broader in scope than those of common usage.

In *Peace Research around the World* Newcombe provides a detailed description of the main definitions, fundamental studies and theories, and action research during the 1950s and 1960s which laid the foundations of peace research.[18]

Peace studies has been defined as 'entailing the hard purification of scholarship. It may contain an experiential component but it is an academic discipline and is not a form of activist enterprise.'[19] Dunn[20] makes a distinction between peace studies, peace research and peace education. Peace research is concerned with the development and accumulation of knowledge; peace education is concerned with the development of the processes of education in and about peace; and peace studies, as an area of concern, relates to the substantive issues regarding the purposes and problems of the dissemination of knowledge of peace as a process. Dunn adds a corollary that, for many people, these distinctions are artificial and unnecessary and, as mentioned previously, the terms are used interchangeably. The role of academic institutions in teaching, studying and researching peace is to provide information and intellectual resources for activists, from which applied methods of pursuing peace can be developed by the peace movement.[21]

The interplay between academic and activist is vital if the peace movement is to remain a dynamic force with any real hope of influencing decision makers; of changing society; and of furthering its aims and objectives. Useful discussions on the theoretical, historical and organisational backgrounds of peace research can be found in Mack,[22] Wilson,[23] Young[24] and Dedring.[25]

Medical peace research has contributed, both from individual and organisational perspectives, to the emerging disciplines of 'conflict studies' and peace research in general. Psychologists and psychiatrists, in particular, have traditionally been involved in studying the etiology and prevention of war, whilst other health professionals have detailed the medical consequences of both nuclear and conventional war. Some examples of their work will be illustrated later in the text.

PHYSICIANS, WAR AND PEACE

Physicians have not always been concerned with the issues mentioned above, or even concerned with providing humanitarian aid to the casualties of war.

In the early Middle Ages the only regular medical provision for the sick and wounded was made by the church, who were translating some of the established Arabic medical treatises into Latin. (Many texts on the history of medicine are available, but a very readable account may be found in *The Relation of Medicine to Philosophy* by R. O. Moon.[26] At the time of the Crusades organisations such as the Knights of St John (1099) and the Teutonic Knights (1200) undertook the nursing care of both soldiers and civilians. The fifteenth century saw barber-surgeons being employed by wealthy soldier-patrons in time of war. If captured by the enemy they readily changed allegiance, and thought of themslves rather like 'medical mercenaries'. However, army service had its disadvantages – if a wealthy, influential patient died under their ministrations, there was danger of mutilation. As a result, these barber-surgeons often had to be conscripted into service. By the time of the seventeenth and eighteenth centuries embryonic state medical hospitals for the army had been established and the beginnings of organised military medical services took root. But care of the wounded and sick was still of a very basic and haphazard nature[27] and medical personnel and the victims of conflict (both civilian and military) had no particular rights of protection. Doctors viewed war as a useful experience in furthering their surgical skills and were not usually concerned with its causes or the resulting devastation.

The Red Cross

A major step in the organisation of medical expertise for humanitarian goals in warfare was taken by Henri Dunant in 1863 with the formation, in Switzerland, of the International Committee for the Relief of the Wounded, which was later to become the International Committee of the Red Cross (ICRC). The ICRC was originally conceived and organised for the purpose of assisting the victims of armed conflicts, without seeking to avoid the conflicts themselves. Dunant wrote: 'if war is unavoidable, then it should be waged with as little barbarity as possible.'[28] On 22 August 1864 the First Geneva Convention was signed for the 'Amelioration of the Condition of the Wounded and Sick in the Armed Forces in the Field'. This convention marked the appearance of International Humanitarian Law (IHL) as a new branch of International Public Law – which aimed to protect the victims of armed conflict and the personnel responsible for taking care of them.[29, 30] Physicians and other defined medical personnel have particular rights and duties incumbent upon them and granted to them by the provisions of IHL, specifically the right of respect and protection. In times of armed conflict they are duty bound to abstain from all acts of hostility; to respect the principles of medical ethics in the same manner as in peacetime; to provide care without any distinction based on other than medical criteria; and are subject to punishment if they commit abuses or breaches of IHL. These provisions are fully described in the *Manual on the Rights and Duties of Medical Personnel in Armed Conflicts*.[31] Medical teams are seen as *neutral* by states who are party to the Geneva Conventions. Three other conventions (and several protocols) have since been added, covering the treatment of prisoners of war, shipwrecked members of armed forces, and the protection of civilians in time of war and national emergencies.[32]

As a result of its humanitarian and impartial action, the ICRC claims to have made an important contribution to peace and humanitarian mediation through its involvement in conflicts internationally.[33, 34, 35]

Social, Political and Ethical Responsibilities

> Physicians should be responsible for the environment in which medical care takes place. They are to be 'healers of social as well as individual pathology'.[36]
>
> As physicians we may identify with the social forces for progress, national and international, and still be among our colleagues. To do so requires some independence of thought and action. Certainly it is in keeping with the role of the physician as an innovator in the health field and as a healer of social as well as individual pathology.[37]

Doctors are citizens and as such have the same social and political responsibilities that are incumbent on all citizens. Do physicians have any particular skills or knowledge, over and above that of other citizens, which can be brought to bear on political and social questions? Physicians in the nineteenth century began to realise that much of human disease was linked to social factors such as poor housing, inadequate sanitation, malnutrition, unsafe working practices, poor education and so on. Far-sighted physicians (such as Rudolph Virchow whose activities will be exampled later) became known not only for their medical expertise but also for their political engagement in agitating for an improvement in the quality of life for all people. Other physicians (like Charles Richet and Albert Skarvan) made the direct connection between the enormous amounts being spent on armaments and war preparations and the inadequate commitment of governments to public health measures. These physicians began a tradition of concern with broader social responsibilities, which are now accepted by many as a core element of the professional roles of health care workers. Peace is a fundamental requirement to enable the achievement of health for all.

Jonsen and Jameton ask the questions: in what sense do physicians have broader social and political responsibilities? and, if they do have them, how is a conflict of responsibilities dealt with? They distinguish between:

- responsibilities to patients
- social responsibilities contingent upon patient responsibilities
- social and political responsibilities beyond patient responsibilities.

The position with regard to patients and colleagues, ethically speaking, is relatively clear. It is the doctor – society relationship which causes the most difficulty and forms a basis for disagreement. There is no reason why the status of doctor should put a citizen in a class of his own ...

> What is, however, more likely, is that the special skills and responsibilities of the medical profession highlight the moral dilemmas of doctors – the dilemmas are more obvious and more frequent than for most other citizens, but the moral laws applying to doctors are the same as for all citizens.[38]

What physicians should do wherever possible is to combat, by taking appropriate social and political action, the immoral application of their skills. Examples of failure to do this are, sadly, many. A particular example, the sour taste of which still lingers, is the manner in which some members of the German medical profession co-operated with the Nazi regime during the 1930s and 1940s. More recently, however, there are examples of physicians refusing to co-operate with war preparations and activities. During the time of the Vietnam War some American physicians refused to train paramedics for the army, and also actively engaged in the facilitation of draft deferments on grounds of physical disability.[39]

Cassel *et al.*[40] were quite clear when they put forward their argument for the involvement of physicians in the prevention of nuclear war. They claimed that nuclear war would cause unprecedented human death and suffering, that physicians have a central moral responsibility to relieve suffering, that public education by physicians could help prevent a nuclear war, and that physicians therefore have a responsibility to work to prevent nuclear war. Later McCally and Cassel[41] extended this argument to compel physicians to add concern for global environmental change to their efforts to reduce the threat of nuclear war. They stress:

> When physicians have special knowledge of dangers to health that are not generally available to others, they have a duty to inform those concerned...

and,

> Health hazards cannot be ruled out as medical concerns because their remedy requires political action.[42]

This view is supported by Lown[43] who says that physicians must respond to the moral imperatives of their commitment to life and health rather than worry about crossing the ill-defined boundary of the political realm.

A word of warning is sounded by Relman in this matter. Writing in the *New England Journal of Medicine*[44] he voiced a concern that if physicians spoke out, as physicians rather than citizens, on controversial public issues (like nuclear disarmament), in which they had no special political competence and about which they are probably as divided as the rest of the citizenry, then they risked losing the confidence of their fellow citizens in their professional competence, thus jeopardising the 'solidarity of their profession'. In other words, it was one thing sounding the warning, but quite another entering the political arena. Relman concludes:

> ... difference of physicians as *citizens* ... what they should not do is confuse personal conviction with professional expertise or make the dangerous assumption that medical professional societies have any special competence or authority in dealing with purely political problems.[45]

Physicians have social, political and moral obligations to become informed and engage themselves in matters which concern the health of their patients. These concerns range from informing the public about the dangers of smoking, about an unhealthy diet, about the danger from asbestos in building materials, through to the ultimate dangers of nuclear war and degradation of the environment. It seems that physicians as a class have shown little interest in political activities unless political and social situations have directly affected them, but the intricate connections between social conditions and the health of individuals are becoming better understood and more widely appreciated.[46] To combat effectively the danger to their patients, and to global society generally, from the consequences of modern, highly destructive means of warfare, the imperatives of sound preventive community medicine must be employed. Physicians in the medical peace movement believe that it is just not good enough to wait for disasters to strike (what point the infinite care taken over a premature baby when these efforts, multiplied many times throughout the world, can be snuffed out in a few seconds?), but believe they should act to empower people to work positively for peace. Their dedication to human health and well-being imposes this responsibility on them. Underlying all these considerations is the primary moral reponsibility of physicians to the due care and personal concern of their patients – at the centre of physicians' responsibilities is the diagnosis and treatment of disease.

CONCLUSION

Doctors have a common set of ethics embodied in such documents as the Hippocratic Oath and the Declaration of Geneva[47, 48] which dedicate their skills to the best interest of their patient. They are morally bound not to participate in the torture or mistreatment of prisoners or patients. It is assumed by many that physicians will not use their professional skills to aid in the wilful or premeditated killing of fellow human beings. Unfortunately, in the real world, physicians can behave in the same debased manner as anybody else and there are many recorded instances of health professionals participating in abuses of basic human rights and dignity.[49]

This book, however, is about those physicians who have striven, and continue to do so, to uphold and work for peace and justice within the true healing spirit of their profession, or as R.O. Moon writes:

> To preserve life must ever be the honour and duty of the physician, but to make life livable should be his aim also.[50]

PART TWO: 1815–1918

PIONEER CITIZEN DIPLOMATS

Towards the end of the eighteenth century two American physicians, Benjamin Rush and George Logan, took individual action in promoting peace processes.

Benjamin Rush

In 1790 Dr Benjamin Rush (1745–1813), who was a signatory of the American Declaration of Independence in 1776, proposed a Peace Department for that country. The first article of the project stated:

> Let a Secretary of the Peace be appointed to preside at this office, who shall be perfectly free from all the present absurd and vulgar European prejudices on the subject of government: Let him be a genuine republican and a sincere Christian, for the principles of republicanism and Christianity are no less friendly to universal and perpetual peace than they are to universal and equal liberty.

Rush, who had served in the War of Independence (1776–83) as an army surgeon and was well aware of the human suffering caused by this violent conflict, adds a corollary to his first article:

> In order the more deeply to affect the minds of the citizens of the United States with the blessings of peace, by contrasting them with the evils of war, let the following inscriptions be painted on the sign which is placed over the door of the war offices:–
>
> 1. An office for butchering the human species.
> 2. A widow and orphan making office.
> 3. A broken bone making office.

4. A wooden leg making office.
5. An office for creating public and private vices.
6. An office for creating public debt.
7. An office for creating speculators, stock jobbers and bankrupts.
8. An office for creating famine.
9. An office for creating political diseases.
10. An office for creating poverty and the destruction of liberty and national happiness.

In the lobby of this office let there be painted representations of all the common military instruments of death; also human skulls, broken bones, unburied and putrefying dead bodies, hospitals crowded with sick and wounded soldiers, villages on fire, mothers in besieged towns eating the flesh of their children, ships sinking in the ocean, rivers dyed with blood, and extensive plains without tree or fence, or any other object but the ruins of deserted farm houses. Above all this group of woeful figures, let the following words be inserted in red characters, to represent human blood:–

NATIONAL GLORY[1]

Benjamin Rush was born into a strict Presbyterian family with emphasis on the importance of a puritanical devotion to moral and religious values – these were of deep significance throughout his life. After completing his medical degree at Princeton University, Rush travelled to Edinburgh where he studied under Joseph Black and William Cullen. Two years later, in 1768, he received his MD. Whilst at Edinburgh he was introduced to republican principles by John Bostock, a fellow medical student, and Catherine Macaulay who was a radical, republican English historian.[2] Rush then travelled to London to continue his studies at St Thomas's Hospital. Whilst in London he met Benjamin Franklin[3] and this friendship further committed him to the republican cause.

Following his return to Philadelphia in late 1768, in addition to his professional work as a medical professor at the University, Rush also became a prominent member of the republican circles of that time. He began to feel more keenly that the decline in moral standards was due mostly to the corrupting influence of English society. In 1773 he published *An Address to the Inhabitants of the British Settlements in America, upon Slave-keeping* and in 1774 helped to organise the Pennsylvania Society for Promoting the Abolition of Slavery. He became closely associated with other independence leaders such as Thomas Jefferson, John Adams and Thomas Paine. Rush had a great influence on the production and publication of *Common Sense*, written by Paine in 1776,[4] having persuaded Paine to write the pamphlet and suggested the title. As a result of his republican anti-English sympathies he was made a member of the Continental Congress and thus on 2 August 1776 signed the American Declaration of Independence. Rush saw the American revolution not only as bringing freedom from England, but also as heralding in a new era:

> . . .which would be notable for its domestic tranquility and for its economic prosperity. Its citizens would be renowned for virtue, piety, and patriotism. Vice would be eliminated . . .especially the sins of idleness and greed. Furthermore, virtually all men would be intelligent voters, knowledgeable on local, state and national issues. Political parties would not exist, for Americans would endeavour to serve their country rather than the particular interest of a group or faction.[5]

He believed that religion was necessary to promote virtue and discourage vice. In 1778 he supported the proposed US Constitution and, believing very strongly in the need for 'checks and balances' in such a document, approvingly noted that 'neither the House of Representatives, the Senate or the President can perform a single legislative act by themselves'.[6]

During the 1790s Rush's medical and political careers came under attack. During 1793 and 1797 there were two serious outbreaks of yellow fever in Philadelphia. Rush was a great advocate of purging or bleeding and in some cases would remove as much as four-fifths of a patient's blood.[7] William Cobbett, a pro-English monarchist immigrant and virulent critic of Rush's, tried to point out the correlation, as he saw it, between the increasing employment of Rush's treatment and the increasing mortality rate – the more bleeding, the more deaths! The doctor's system, Cobbett observed, is 'one of the great discoveries . . . which have contributed to the depopulation of the earth'.[8]

By 1800 Rush was disenchanted with American society. He saw the 'worshipping' of George Washington as significant evidence of a corrupt society and considered the new economic system, involving 'speculators' and a general 'lust' after money, un-republican: good republicans were productive and frugal. The war of 1812 with England gave rise to more disillusionment, particularly as Rush saw that many citizens did not support the war effort to protect their rights and independence. For him:

> . . . a field of battle covered with dead bodies was not so awful a spectacle as a nation deliberately preferring slavery to liberty, and commerce to national independence.[9]

Bearing in mind his Peace Department proposal of 1790 this seems a little incongruous. Throughout his life Rush retained his pious outlook which had been instilled in him during his early years. His occasional use of theological arguments in medical reasoning was a survival of medievalism in method entirely foreign to his contemporaries.[10]

But Rush began a tradition of involvement, by American physicians, in social and political issues which continues today. His activities in the areas of prison reform, abolition of slavery, improved education for women (he also founded the Presbyterian Dickinson College), compassionate treatment of the insane and a sincere belief in peace and justice reflected the thinking of 'radical' liberal concerns of his time.

George Logan and Mediation

Also active in Pennsylvania at this time was Dr George Logan (1753–1821). Like Benjamin Rush he too studied medicine at Edinburgh (graduating ten years after Rush in 1779) and also met and was influenced by the republican ideals of Benjamin Franklin, whom he was introduced to whilst studying anatomy in Paris during 1780. This friendship lasted until the latter's death.[11]

Logan grew up in a strict Quaker family, although he did not adhere to the Quakers' 'conscientious objection' to all war, believing instead that Christian proscription against war did not include conflicts 'strictly of a defensive kind'.[12] (This thinking caused a rift between Logan and the Philadelphian Quakers when he joined the Pennsylvanian Militia in

1791.) On his return from Paris in 1780, due to the death of his father and brother, he inherited the family farm, and from then on he devoted much of his time to farming. He was a fervent Jeffersonian republican and advocated public education, negro emancipation and dominance of agriculture over industry.[13]

In 1798 Logan undertook a one-man peace mission to France in an attempt to end the undeclared naval war between France and the US. Armed with a letter of introduction from Jefferson, he sailed to France and managed to meet Talleyrand and other French officials.[14] As a consequence of his visit some captured American seamen were released, France agreed to lift an embargo on US ships, and also agreed to welcome a US envoy. Back home in America a hostile Congress greeted him. The federalists managed to get Congress to pass the Logan Act in 1799. This made it illegal for a private citizen to undertake diplomatic missions without official sanction. President John Adams was more friendly and Logan's initiative supplemented information he had received from other sources. This encouraged him to persist in seeking a peaceful outcome to the crisis. Logan's public standing was enhanced and he was elected to the Senate in 1801.

In 1810, disregarding the Logan Act, he went to Britain in an unsuccessful attempt to halt the drift towards war between the two countries, which eventually erupted in 1812. George Logan's success in ignoring the punitive Logan Act underscores American acceptance of a role for private mediatory missions in the conduct of foreign affairs.[15] Whether or not Logan's intervention was the critical factor in freeing the American sailors in France, he served both French and American interests as a conduit for the termination of hostilities.

The Logan Act is still in force today and could have been applied, for example, in preventing the visit of US presidential candidate Jesse Jackson to Damascus, Syria, in 1984. In this private visit he attempted to secure the release of a captured US serviceman.[16]

THE FIRST PEACE SOCIETIES: 1815–43

Before highlighting the contributions to peace by some of the more important personalities and organisations of the medical world, it is useful to present a sketch of the first peace societies.

In America, David Low Dodge formed the world's first Peace Society on 14 August 1815.[17] He denounced all warfare as contrary to Christianity. In Great Britain, a small group of Quakers (who were to play a prominent part in the early days of the peace movement) founded a similar group, 'to consider measures for the promotion of Permanent and Universal Peace', on 14 June 1816. Howard[18] calls this the beginning of what was to become known as 'the Peace Movement'; that is, he says, 'the political organisation of middle-class liberals on a transnational basis to secure, by education, agitation and propaganda, the abolition of war'. The British society was strictly pacifist and advocated non-resistance. Beales[19] noted that many people remained outside the Peace Society on the sole ground of its opposition to defensive war. He identified five fundamental schemes, all interrelated and interdependent, which were the focus of intensive campaigning by the peace societies during the nineteenth century: arbitration, arbitration treaties and clauses in treaties, an International Authority or Tribunal or Congress, the codification of International Law, and disarmament.[20]

In 1829, under the influence of William Ladd, the American Peace Society was formed. This was a consolidation of all the peace societies which had sprung up throughout the US and from the beginning had precise aims, declared in an early circular:

> We hope to increase and promote the practice already begun of submitting national differences to amicable discussion and arbitration; and finally of settling all national controversies by an appeal to reason, as becomes rational creatures . . . and this shall be done by a Congress of Nations, whose decrees shall be enforced by public opinion that rules the world . . . Then wars shall cease.[21]

The proponents of the Free Trade Movement (which started about 1830 with the Industrial Revolution and the resulting rapid development of the transport system) greatly strengthened the peace movement. Men such as Richard Cobden united the causes of free trade and peace, particularly in the European context. For Cobden they were 'one and the same cause'.[22] Both in England and America between 1830 and 1842 much work was done to get the virtues of arbitration discussed in parliaments and recognised by ministers as practical ways of resolving conflicts. The American Peace Society promoted vigorously the idea of a Congress of Nations and prominent Quaker families threw in their support for the peace movement.

By 1843 there was enough support for a first General Peace Convention to be held in London with 324 delegates from America and Europe present; resolutions were passed regarding arbitration, the proposed Congress of Nations, methods of propaganda and so on. A plea was also made for the formation of 'associations among the working classes'.[23] A second Peace Congress was organised in 1848 and they were held annually from then on until 1854, with the outbreak of the Crimean War. The Anglo-American peace movement had begun to decline in 1851. Contributing to the causes of this were several factors:[24]

- Increasing nationalism in Europe and an accelerating arms race.
- Early leaders were ageing, with nobody emerging to take over from them.
- In Europe the Crimean War (1854) and an increasingly hostile press made it difficult for the peace societies to function.
- In America the growing issue of slavery was becoming urgent for peace movement activists. The peace movement was split internally over a basic moral issue: the debate between the absolutists in the movement, who opposed use of violence in the approaching civil war and objected in any case to any involvement in war making, and that faction who saw the resort to war as being morally justified in the fight against slavery. *This dilemma is to recur throughout the history of the peace movement.* On this issue Beales has to say:

> The fatal significance of slavery for the peace movement lay in that the champions of peace were also the prophets of Abolition. A conflict of loyalties arose which could not but wreck at least one of the causes, unless some plausible sophistries could be invented that would simplify the issue and facilitate a decision one way or the other without affronting conscience. Thus in America abolition triumphed over peace on the easy assumption that the conflict was a rebellion (not an international war) and so outside the orbit of the Peace Society; while in England peace triumphed over abolition on the non-resistant argument that *all* war was unchristian and anaethema. The result was disastrous

for the American Peace Society and for amicable relations between the peace advocates of both hemispheres.[25]

Against this background in Europe there were two notable physicians who, during the latter half of the nineteenth century, worked tirelessly for peace, justice and international regulation. Their actions represent thinking about peace and war prevalent at that time amongst medical 'peace' activists. They were Rudolph Virchow and Adolph Fischoff.

DR RUDOLPH VIRCHOW

One of the most outspoken activists of this era in Europe was the German physician Dr Rudolph Virchow (1821–1902), physician, politician and peace worker. After qualifying in Berlin in 1843, Virchow became active in politics of the extreme radical left during the revolutionary struggle for a united Germany.[26] At this time he was the driving force behind the Medical Reform Group and its medico-political journal *Die Medicinische Reform*. This group, with Virchow as its spokesman, believed that medicine, if it is to reduce morbidity and mortality, must attend at one and the same time to the biological *and* to the social roots of disease. Virchow stated:

> Medicine is a social science, and politics is nothing more than medicine on a large scale.
> The improvement of medicine will eventually prolong human life, but the improvement of social conditions can achieve this result more rapidly and more successfully.[27]

Virchow was a consistent critic of Bismarck and the Prussian militaristic philosophy pervasive in Germany at that time. He was a member of the Prussian Landtag (from 1862) and, after the unification of the German State, the Reichstag (from 1880 to 1893). Whilst a member of the Landtag he was challenged to a duel by Bismarck who viewed Virchow's unwilting attacks on his military budget as a personal affront. This was only averted because Bismarck's political associates persuaded him that he would look ridiculous duelling publicly with a *parvenu*.

In 1869 Virchow presented his famous motion on disarmament to the Landtag.[28] In this motion he asked that Prussia take a lead in disarmament and pointed out that expenditures, in that country, for education had remained stationary because military expenditures were consuming an ever-increasing share of the budget. He stressed the process of conflict spiral: '... the size of our army provides a pretence for other countries to strengthen theirs...'[29] This motion, and similar ones throughout Europe, were defeated. Virchow's plea did however receive world-wide publicity. (The following year, in July 1870, the Franco-Prussian War erupted.) Virchow was a tireless fighter for the rights of all and during the 1870s and 1880s he resisted the virulent anti-Semitism, a movement which Bismarck tacitly supported. He refuted the concept of racial purity of the German nation by carrying out a series of investigations between peoples by comparing their anthropometric measurements..

Virchow was in contact with many of Europe's leading pacifists, such as Edmond Potonie-Pierre, whom he encouraged to form the *Ligue du Bien Public* in 1858. This was formed in an attempt to revive the idea of the peace conferences of 1848–51 and, although this aim was not achieved, the *Ligue* formed an important link between the Anglo-American Crusade which was then declining and the Continental Crusade which was to begin around 1865. Virchow was instrumental, with Alfred Fried and others, in the formation of the German Peace Union in 1894 with a membership of 4,000 active members. In 1899 he campaigned for support of the first Hague Peace Conference within Germany.

In addition to being active politically, Virchow was probably the foremost medical scientist of his time. He established cell doctrine in pathology which William Henry Welch was to hail as 'one of the greatest events in the history of medicine'.[30] He contributed to the fields of public health and health education, and helped develop a modern sewage system for Berlin; he continually linked the needs for social justice, human rights and disarmament as prerequisites for a peaceful world. After studying an epidemic of typhus which had broken out in the region of Upper Silesia, 1884, Virchow requested full and unlimited democratic government, free education, raising the standard of living, availability of specialists to help with the treatment, and the improvement of agricultural techniques for the region.[31] In his paper, Eisenberg says of Virchow:

...his courage in speaking out for fundamental human rights provides an example to sustain us at a time when the propriety of what we do here is under attack as a 'misuse' of medicine for political ends.[32]

DR ADOLPH FISCHOFF

Like Virchow, Dr Adolph Fischoff (1816–93) became involved in revolutionary activities after he had qualified. Fischoff graduated in 1845 from the University of Vienna, was soon active in political affairs and was arrested during the 1848 Austrian revolution (he was a liberal advocate of constitutional reform[33]). After his release he combined the practice of medicine with a life in politics and in 1875 published *On the Reduction of Continental Armies*. In this article, which appeared in two parts on 26 and 28 September 1875, in the *Neue freie Presse* (Vienna) he called on the nations of Europe to cease their arms race, halt research and development of new weapons systems, and called for a conference consisting of elected parliamentary representatives and representatives from non-parliamentary countries to discuss disarmament measures. Of the arms race and the general mistrust between the powers he said:

> Governments hardly know who goes first, or who follows after; what is the cause, or what is effect; who is the threatened, or who is the threatener.[34]

A result of such a conference would be better understanding and communication between the governments of Europe. The conference could make two resolutions to help this process:

1. Set a limit on the size of respective armies.
2. For representatives to put a motion before their own parliaments calling on them to reduce their armed forces in accordance with a quota named by the conference, if the other powers would do the same simultaneously. These reductions would be formulated in such a way that the security of any state would not be threatened.[35]

Fischoff felt that diplomats had failed, and would continue to fail, to make any real progress in disarmament and arbitration issues because of the vested interests they served. There was too much enmity within Europe at this time (particularly between France and Prussia after the 1870 war) for his idea to take hold. Peace proposals were generally viewed as being utopian and most reform groups at this time were more concerned with women's suffrage and the abolition of slavery.

In proposing real cuts in military budgets he wrote:

> The reduction of war estimates is not a remedy that proves effectual, if applied in infinitesimal homoeopathic doses. From the depths of its sufferings, Europe calls open-mouthed for a strong dose of this particular medicine. The hand which applies it must neither halt nor hesitate. A council of medical assessors must therefore watch over it, in order that there may be no wavering, no half measures, and no neglect.[36]

Fischoff was the foremost pacifist in Austria and his ideas and leadership stimulated the formation of the Austrian Peace Society of 1889 as well as the Interparliamentary Union of the same year. He thought that world government, international arbitration and mutually balanced arms reductions were the practical ways forward to secure a peaceful world.

SOCIALIST AND FEMINIST INFLUENCES

The first Socialist International (also known as the International Working Men's Association) was established in 1864. Under the influence of Karl Marx it distrusted collaboration with any middle-class organisation, even on a cross-class issue such as peace. It took the position that war resulted from capitalist exploitation and, therefore, that peace would be the natural product of the socialist revolution. It also refused to permit the participation of women.[37]

Two women physicians, Dr Anna Kulisciolf (1854–1925) and Dr Madeleine Pelletier (1874–1939), were particularly active in Continental Europe at this time with regard to peace, and feminist and socialist concerns.

Anna Kuliscioff was born in Kherson, Russia, in 1854. In 1871 she left her home for the University of Zurich to study engineering, since this course of study was closed to women in Russia at that time. Whilst in Switzerland she lived with, but did not marry, the Italian anarchist Andrea Costa and had a daughter by him. Active in Anarchist International (she was a supporter of Bakunin), she was arrested in Florence in 1878 during a government crackdown on anarchists, held in 'preventive imprisonment' for 14 months, then tried and acquitted of a charge of conspiring against the state. Soon after her return to Switzerland the relationship with Costa ended, and in 1882 she entered the University of Berne to study medicine. In 1884 she moved to the University of Naples from where she graduated as a doctor in 1886. She set up practice in Milan, specialising in gynaecology. Before finishing her medical studies she had left the anarchists (in 1885) and become a lifelong committed Marxist.[38]

The letters of Anna Kuliscioff to the Marxist Filippo Turati[39] (who was the co-founder with her of the Italian Socialist Party [PSI]) illustrate the strong connection between European Socialism and the peace movement before the First World War. These letters reveal Kuliscioff's twofold approach to peace from her socialist standpoint. First, she supported the Zurich Congress of the Second International in 1893, that is, that once European workers understood that the working class was united by strong bonds of mutual self-esteem against the world's capitalists, it would no longer be possible for the bourgeois governments to use nationalism to turn workers into soldiers. Without soldiers there could be no war. Second, she encouraged socialists in the Italian Parliament in their efforts to trim the military budget to the minimum necessary for defence, so freeing funds for social programmes. The Italian military establishment was denounced for squandering the country's wealth, for perpetuating societal inequities, and for holding the prevention of revolution rather than national defence as its main goal. But Kuliscioff and Turati argued against prevalent socialist demands that Italy disarm unilaterally on the grounds that it was simplistic and impractical.[40]

Along with the liberals and radicals, the socialists identified the arms race as one of the main threats to peace. Blame was laid at the feet of private armament firms and arms traders over whom more control was needed. Cooper notes that from its origins the Italian peace movement had always sought closer ties and collaboration with organised socialist groups such as the PSI.[41]

Kuliscioff was also an active feminist and her two commitments – to feminism and Marxism – often clashed. Women, the sex defended by feminists, cut vertical lines through society and this included female capitalists, the exploiters of proletarian men and women. The proletariat, the class championed by the Marxists, cut horizontally across society and therefore included men, the exploiters of women.[42] Her thinking on these issues was laid out in *The Monopoly of the Male* (1890), in which these two strands in her life were discussed.[43] However, with the formation of the PSI in 1892, socialism became the dominant influence. Devotion to the cause of the pure ideal, the proletariat, was doubtless easier than devotion to the women with whom she worked and whom she deemed chatty, unreliable and empty-headed.[44]

In 1912 Kuliscioff and Turati lost control of the PSI to a rival revolutionary faction led by Benito Mussolini and from then on Kulisioff concentrated on the issue of women's suffrage. Before Italy entered the First World War, in May 1915, there had been much debate in socialist circles on what should be done in the event of war: would individual socialists support the International or their respective national war efforts? (This was a debate mirrored in other European countries at that time.) In 1915 the PSI was almost isolated with its policy of passive opposition to the war, most of the other peace groups supporting Italy's entry. Kulisicoff promoted PSI's slogan 'neither support nor sabotage', and her anti-war principles held firm until October 1917 when the Germans broke the line at Caporetto and nationalism swayed her to urge Turati and the PSI to support the war effort.[45]

Madeleine Pelletier, unlike Kulisicoff, did break with the revolutionary socialists over women's suffrage. Pelletier had been elected to the central administrative committee of the revolutionary socialists which would have transferred power to the workers, but she feared that this would only enshrine the traditional restrictions (of women) under a new name. 'The working class,' she predicted, 'will be the last to accept feminism. The ignorant respect nothing but brute force.'[46] She linked war with anti-feminism, calling it the basis of men's power over women.[47] By the outbreak of the First World War she had concluded that the left wing had nothing to offer women. The French socialists dismissed reforms proposed by feminists as bourgeois or premature – women could only practise socialism by rejecting feminism.[48]

Pelletier believed that war was a learned behaviour – if boys were not given wooden rifles, they would not dream of becoming soldiers. She also thought that because women were not prepared for war, women's suffrage represented a powerful means of combating militarism. Pelletier, like Kuliscioff, felt betrayed by the socialists who supported the war. However, she did attempt to join the medical corps and, when she failed, volunteered for the Red Cross, in which she served from 1915 on the front line and where, to the horror of her comrades, she treated the wounded of both sides.[49] The same dilemma had confronted French socialists as well as Italians with the coming of war in 1914. According to Charles Chatfield, 'widespread socialist support for WW1 contravened pre-war expressions of international workers' solidarity; but it reflected the pragmatic and nationalistic elements in socialist thought'.[50]

By 1925 Pelletier, the Internationalist, was disillusioned with collective action and concentrated full-time on her medical practice, treating the exhausted wives of workers, 'administered first a blow and then a baby' by drunken husbands.[51] At the age of 64 she was committed to an asylum for performing abortions on the poor women with whom she was working. She died six months later.

ALBERT SKARVAN'S ACT OF INDIVIDUAL DEFIANCE

The witness for peace of Dr Albert Skarvan (1869–1926) was not a result of political motivation but due to the influence of Leo Tolstoy.[52] It was in 1895 that Skarvan, a surgeon in the Slovak army, refused, a few weeks before he was due to finish his term of service in the army, to continue to serve any longer. After reading Tolstoy, he was convinced that the practice of Christianity precluded any association with the machinery of war.[53] As a result he was imprisoned. On his release he travelled to Russia where he met Tolstoy and befriended Dr Dusan Makovicky, Tolstoy's physician. After exile in England and Switzerland he was allowed to return home in 1910, when he took up practice as a country doctor. No large-scale anti-war movement happened as a reuslt of Tolstoy's teachings, but Skarvan, until his death in 1926, continued to advocate non-violence and to regard the state as unChristian. For the peace movement his importance lies in his act of individual defiance, as a conscientious objector, to the Austro-Hungarian authorities.[54]

Up until now the work of individual physicians, for the most part working from a political context, has been looked at. In France the first solely medical international group was formed in 1905 to protest against war and war preparations.

INTERNATIONAL MEDICAL ASSOCIATION AGAINST WAR (IMAW)

In March 1905, in the midst of the Russo-Japanese War, the French physician, Joseph Rivière (1859–1946), sent a circular to a certain number of his medical friends, French and foreign, stating:

> The horrors of the present war have suggested to several colleagues as well as myself, the idea of assembling at Paris . . . an International Congress of medical men, who in the name of their mission to humanity, would meet to protest against armed conflicts, thus bringing a powerful assistance to the work of peace by arbitration.[55]

As a result of this, a meeting was held at Rivière's home and the *Association médicale Internationale contre la guerre* was formed on 21 March.[56] Officers were appointed and statutes of the associations drawn up.[57] These included:

Art. 2. The basis of the Association is respect of human life, its aim the abolition of war.

Art. 3. The Association proposes to rally the medical men of the whole world in view of permanent protestation against war, and in view of creating a current of ideas, feelings and opinions against all armed conflicts.

Art. 4. The Association is exclusively composed of medical men.

The IMAW also hoped to organise an International Congress every third year. Rivière was elected President and under his energetic direction the Association grew rapidly. By 1910 it had members in 41 countries[58] and membership lists included 268 members in France, 131 in Italy, 60 in Great Britain[59], 57 in Spain, 51 in the US, 46 in Russia, etc. Alfred Fried in his *Handbook of the Peace Movement* (published 1911–13) reported that the Association had 6,000 members.[60] By 1908

IMAW was an integral part of the peace movement of the day and participated fully in the 17th Universal Congress of Peace held in London that year. At the Congress[61] Rivière and IMAW argued that international disputes should be settled by two tribunals, based at The Hague. The first, an International Tribunal, would form an opinion and deliver a judgement on international questions, and the second, a Humanitarian Tribunal, would have supreme jurisdiction on all matters. They considered that the moral force of these two tribunals, backed up if necessary by an international constabulary, would be sufficient to ensure real justice. Rivière also talked of his concern over the effect that violence, in the then rapidly developing film industry, might have on younger people and he also supported the idea of 'peace education' in schools. Rivière and IMAW supported the ideas of the Free Trade Movement and stated:

> Until all peoples have come to understand the benefits of free trade, which would be enough in itself to do away with the causes of modern wars, we are of the opinion that, in order to abolish warfare, it would be sufficient, in the meanwhile, to apply to nations the laws which govern individuals.[62]

The IMAW continued campaigning for their aims up to the outbreak of the First World War. With the beginning of hostilities Rivière offered his services to treat the wounded and the activities of IMAW ceased. His medical skills at this time earned him honours from the French, Canadian and American governments. With the end of the war, Rivière again took up campaigning for international arbitration. He gave much attention to the importance, as he saw it, of French–American friendship, and lobbied hard for American support of the League of Nations. During the 1920s he toured the US extensively, lecturing on his medical speciality, physicotherapy,[63] and peace. The *Atlanta Georgian* of 14 January 1926 recorded a speech delivered by him at Salt Lake City, Utah, in which he spoke, however, against disarmament at that time. This reflected his views on what he saw as a threat from the Bolsheviks:

> I have spent my life in an effort to prevent war, but to disarm before there is a Union of Nations functioning as successfully as the Union of States in America is like putting the cart before the

horse... cancer cells are like Bolsheviks of the human body... and Anarchists, more horrible and treacherous than Red Russians, are also cancer cells.

Joseph Rivière died in 1946, a successful and respected physician. His thinking strongly reflected the views of his time which tended to be legalistic and moral in tone – it was argued that the future of world peace depended on institutions such as the League of Nations and International Tribunals. IMAW can be seen as a true precursor of International Physicians for the Prevention of War (IPPNW)[64] and its success was due mostly to the personal efforts of Rivière. He should be recognised as one of the eminent figures in the history of the medical peace movement.

CHARLES RICHET AND IDIOT MAN

Reference has already been made to Professor Charles Richet (1850–1935) of the Faculty of Medicine, University of Paris, who was awarded the Nobel Peace Prize for Physiology in 1913 for his work on anaphylaxis. Like Rivière, Richet was an internationalist and became President of the French Society for International Arbitration which had been founded by Frederic Passy. He attended many national and international peace conferences and worked both with the Carnegie Endowment for International Peace and the International Peace Bureau. In 1900 he presided over the Universal Peace Congress in Paris, regarded as the most successful meeting of that group.[65] Richet linked the spending on armaments of the major powers to the deficiencies in scientific research, cultural activities and the plight of the poor and working class. His writings and speeches also attacked the extreme nationalists and the so-called realists who insisted that high military expenditure assured national security. His pen attacked false patriotism and twisted social Darwinism.[66]

The outbreak of the First World War was a bitter psychological blow to Richet. He volunteered his medical services and was instrumental in developing transfusion techniques which saved the lives of many frontline soldiers. Here he witnessed the full futility and horror of 'modern' warfare. His response to his experiences was a book, *L'Homme Stupide*,[67] published in 1919. In it he wrote that we should forget the classification Linnaeus gave us – *Homo sapiens* or Wise (Thinking) Man – and call ourselves *Homo stultus* or Stupid (Idiot) Man. He lists many examples of what he considered man's foolish habits and superstitions such as the custom of mutilations, clashes between different races, the continuing social evils of drug and alcohol abuse, the spread of venereal disease and syphilis, the wanton destruction of rainforests and man's pointless cruelty to animals.

For him war was a contradiction in Darwinist evolutionary terms as he saw them. Instead of the best of the species being selected for survival:

> War wipes out the young, the strong, the brave leaving only the sweepings and scum of humanity for women to mate with for the protection of the species.[68]

Hope rested in the improvement of human intelligence by selective 'breeding and mating of the fittest'. Richet believed that better communication between nations was vital and to that end supported the teaching of Esperanto (see below) as the universal language. Writing about man's destruction of the environment by war and pollution, he said:

> ... hounded on by the lust of destruction, the human race will make a desert around itself. Certainly men will ultimately rule, but it will be an inglorious reign over a world despoiled of beauty...[69]

In the terms of today's nuclear warfare, Richet's *L'Homme Stupide* would not even have this satisfaction. Although he continued to work for international organisation after the war, Richet was disillusioned and his expectations of what could be done were far more limited.

OTHER PHYSICIAN PACIFISTS ACTIVE BEFORE THE FIRST WORLD WAR

We have already mentioned Esperanto. This language was invented by Dr Ludwik Zamenhof (1859–1917) who completed his medical studies at the University of Warsaw in 1885. Russian-born Zamenhof was a skilled linguist who felt that international peace and understanding would be furthered if all the peoples of the world could speak a common language. To this end he invented Esperanto,[70] a new language which is still studied today.

Concerns about peace were being aired in medical congresses in the years before the First World War. In 1912 an international congress of gynaecologists took place in Berlin. One of the most remarkable speeches was that by the official representative of the Austrian Government, Privy Counsellor Professor Dr Friedrich Schauta. He said:

> Today the palm of victory no longer belongs to that nation which knows best how to conduct war, but to that nation which knows best how to avoid war and preserve the peace. The pride of civilised states in our time is no longer to be found in the destruction of the greatest possible number of individuals, but, on the contrary, they find it in their preservation. In this goal modern medicine, especially modern gynaecology, and the modern civilised states join hands together.[71]

In his *Handbuch der Friedensbewegung* Fried[72] gives some brief details of other physicians who were active in the peace movement before the First World War. From Sweden, Dr Nils August Nilsson was President of the Swedish Peace and Arbitration League (1900–05); founder and President of the Swedish Peace Union/League (1905–10); member of the International Peace Bureau and editor of the peace journal *Svensk Fredstidning* between 1905 and 1909. He lectured energetically throughout Sweden, Norway and Denmark and attended many of the World and Nordic Peace Congresses of that time. He appears to have been one of the main driving forces in the Swedish peace movement of the decade leading up to the First World War.

In Poland, Dr J. Polak, who was a member of the Council of State and an adviser to Warsaw City Council on public health matters, founded (1906), and presided over, the Polish Peace Society. In his *A Short Contribution to the History of Pacifism in Poland*[73] Polak describes how this 'Polish Association of the Friends of Peace' was formed with much advice from Bertha Suttner, probably the leading

European pacifist of that time. He helped popularise the idea of 'peace' through meetings and conferences and articles in the Polish press. Also active internationally, he was vice-president of the 1908 London Peace Congress, which Joseph Rivière attended and where the IMAW were well represented.

Dr Henri Monnier was promoting peace in Switzerland where he was a member of the central committee of the Swiss Peace Society and co-editor of the pacifist organ of Swiss Romansch.

Not all pacifist action stopped with the outbreak of the First World War, as we shall now see.

THE FIRST WORLD WAR (1914–18)

At the outbreak of the First World War the peace movement struggled to survive. Outside its ranks it met with suspicion and contempt, with the charge of 'defeatism', and in most countries with ruthless suppression.[74] Organisations with their bases in neutral countries, such as the International Peace Bureau in Berne, did manage to survive. In Britain some activity continued with the National Peace Council co-ordinating any remaining sections of the peace movement. In October 1914 the Union of Democratic Control (UDC) was founded by E.D. Morel, Norman Angell (whose pamphlet *The Great Illusion* caused so much controversy) and others. It was not a peace society or stop-the-war movement as such, but had the aim of working out bases for lasting peace. Morel, whose watchwords were Native Rights, Freedom of Trade, and Open Diplomacy, was eventually imprisoned in 1917 for contravening the Defence of the Realm Act.[75] The UDC opposed encroachments of 'Prussianism' on British life, in particular the degree to which the methods of the enemy were being copied in the conflict, that is, censorship, compulsion and regimentation.[76] To combat the Conscription Act of 1914 (Great Britain), Fenner Brockway, Bertrand Russell, Clifford Allen and others framed the No Conscription Fellowship (NCF). The main aim of the NCF was the 'removal of conscription from the life of the country of free tradition', and only secondarily opposition to the war as such.[77]

In 1917 a coalition of churches (Baptists, United Free Church and Methodists) formed a United Peace Fellowship (UPF) with the common platform of 'peace by conciliation'. The UPF obtained its inspiration from the principle that war and the preparation for war are contrary to the spirit and teaching of Jesus Christ. One of the most influential religious pacifist groups was the Fellowship of Reconciliation initiated by Dr Henry Hodgkin.

FELLOWSHIP OF RECONCILIATION

Dr Henry Hodgkin (1877–1933) was a Quaker medical missionary with extensive experience of working in China. Hodgkin was spurred into action at the outbreak of the First World War when he realised that many of his close friends on the Continent were officially about to become his 'enemies'. During the last few days of 1914 he called a meeting of 130 Christian pacifists at Cambridge to form the Fellowship of Reconciliation (FOR), a non-sectarian body of individuals dedicated to promoting a spirit of Christian reconciliation.[78] The word 'reconciliation' was chosen to suggest that peace was much more than the absence of war. It was a method of waging war on war – 'the art and practice of turning enemies into friends'.[79] They drew up a five-point document, later known as 'The Basis',[80] which expressed their common Christian convictions and laid down three general principles:

1. That the Fellowship would work constructively for reconciliation, and not spend its energies in mere protest.
2. That its purpose was to bring into being a new order based on Christian principles.
3. That members should work out the implications of membership in their own lives, and not be tied to a stereotyped programme.

Members of FOR showed considerable courage in embracing these principles in wartime since they were viewed with suspicion and, in some cases, were persecuted by officialdom because of their links with the 'enemy' through the network of FOR. Hodgkin remained absolute in his opposition to war and as a conscientious objector he demanded, and received, complete exemption from all wartime service except peace work.[81] After the end of the First World War Hodgkin returned to China as head of the National Christian Council of China and, although not an active member of the peace movement between the two wars, remained committed to the Quaker peace testimony until his death in 1933.

The First World War also stimulated the formation of an international women's peace movement, and we will now look briefly at its origins and activities.

WOMEN MOBILISE AGAINST THE WAR

In April 1915 over 1,100 delegates from 12 countries (including Germany, Belgium, the United States and Great Britain) assembled at The Hague for a congress called by women leaders of various suffrage and social reform movements.[82] The women had decided in advance not to discuss the relative national responsibility for, or the conduct of, the war. The meeting had been convened by Dr Aletta Jacobs (1854–1929), a Dutch physician who had been the first woman in that country to graduate in medicine and who was deeply committed to the campaigns for suffrage and peace.

Resolutions passed at the congress protested the unprecedented human suffering caused by the war; condemned territorial transfers without the consent of the governed; demanded permanent arbitration and mediation to resolve future international conflicts; insisted on democratic control of foreign policy and on women's right to vote. The congress also established an International League for Permanent Peace (ILPP)[83] whose main role was to maintain contact between women pacifists internationally.

Arranging the congress in itself was a considerable achievement given the nationalistic, pro-war feelings generally prevalent at that time, and the obstacles from various belligerent European governments. To help publicise the resolutions passed by the congress, a bold plan was decided upon. Two delegations were organised, to present in person the women's plan for peace to various world leaders. The first, consisting of Aletta Jacobs and Jane Addams (a pioneering social worker from the US), visited the political leaders of the warring countries, while a similar group visited the neutrals. Accompanying Jacobs and Addams was another woman physician, Dr Alice Hamilton (1869–1970),[84] who worked closely with Addams in the US and looked after her health. At The Hague congress she had spoken on the medical consequences of war. (Later, however, when the US entered the war in 1917, Hamilton ceased being a vocal opponent for fear that her peace activities would result in the loss of her job with the US Department of

Labour.⁸⁵) The visits proved very successful and convinced the women that the plan of starting mediation through a continuous conference of the neutral nations was a serious possibility, entertained by both belligerents and neutrals.⁸⁶

In 1915 Jacobs travelled to the US and met President Wilson to pass on an offer from the Dutch Prime Minister that Holland would be willing to call a conference of neutral countries in case Wilson himself was reluctant to do so. Although the President listened carefully to the proposal, nothing came of it. Whilst Jacobs was in the US she was interviewed by Crystal Benedict who was then vice-chairman of the Women's Peace Party of New York. Jacobs made the following observations:

> ... women must show that when all Europe seems full of hatred they can remain united... woman suffrage and permanent peace will go together ... yes the women will do it [vote for peace]. They don't feel as men do about war. They are the mothers of the race.⁸⁷

When asked if women should be represented at a neutral conference of some sort, Jacobs, according to Crystal Benedict, smiled – 'the knowing tolerant smile of a mother for her boys. It made her seem less of a feminist.' Jacobs replied:

> Men, you know, like to do things for themselves. They have more confidence in a proposal if it is made by men than if it is made by women. So, we don't care so very much about having women on the Conference of Neutrals, *if only the right men can be found.*

After the end of the First World War Alice Hamilton worked with the Women's Committee on the Cause and Cure of War which, from 1925 until 1939, campaigned on peace issues in the US and examined the war phenomenon. The work of the committee is reflected in a volume it published in 1935, *Why Wars Must Cease*, to which Hamilton contributed a chapter entitled 'Because War Breeds War'.⁸⁸ Although she retained her pacifist beliefs throughout the 1930s, she was totally opposed to the Nazi regime and supported the Allied war efforts of 1939–45. After the Second World War she criticised the cold war mentality in the US and in 1963 she reaffirmed her pacifism when she signed an open letter protesting the American military involvement in Vietnam.[89]

Around the time of the First World War some physicians and psychologists were trying to understand the causes of war and conflict and it is now appropriate to look at the work of three men who were researching and writing in this area.

MEDICAL THINKING ON THE CAUSES OF WAR

Dr George Friedrich Nicolai (1874–1964): The Tribal Instinct

George Friedrich Nicolai, an eminent cardiologist, was Professor of Physiology at Berlin University when the First World War broke out. He was one of the very few Germans who openly took an anti-war stance from the outset of the conflict. As a result of the uproar created throughout the world after Germany had violated Belgium's neutrality, the Imperial German Government encouraged 93 leading intellectuals (including Ehrlich, Rontgen and von Behring) to sign a public declaration – the 'Manifesto to the Civilised World' – in October 1914. The Manifesto disclaimed German war guilt; denied charges of violation of Belgium's neutrality, asserting that the Germans had merely anticipated the war plans of the Allies and that it would have been suicide to do otherwise; denied German atrocities, specifically the alleged pillage of the Belgian city of Louvain; accused the Allies of using dum-dum bullets; and denounced the 'shameful spectacle . . .of Russians hordes. . . allied with Mongols and Negroes . . . unleashed against the white race'.[90] Within days Nicolai had written a reply – 'Appeal to the Europeans' – and circulated it amongst academic colleagues. Only Albert Einstein and Wilhelm Forster were brave enough to sign it in the charged atmosphere of the time.

In his Appeal, Nicolai explored the rupture of European cultural ties; predicted that there would be no real victors and that all participants would plead for the formation of a League of Europeans to unite the Continent in the cause of peace. Because of a lack of support from his peers Nicolai dropped his Appeal. As a result of this overt anti-war activity he was dismissed from his post, vilified and imprisoned in an old Prussian fortress. During this time he wrote *The Biology of War*, a scientific anti-war treatise which was to become one of the most influential works of its kind in this period.[91] In describing the book Zuelzer writes that:

> Seeking to place pacifism on an objective scientific basis, Nicolai combined biological data and population statistics with historical and cultural arguments to support his thesis that war in the technological age had become an anachronism, analogous to cannibalism and slavery as an obsolete, inefficient, and morally unacceptable means of resolving conflicts of interest between nations.[92]

Nicolai opposed the Social Darwinist apology for war which was prevalent in Germany. The apologists acclaimed the principles of struggle and survival of the fittest as fundamental principles, war being seen as an instrument of evolution and an agent of process in the elimination of the weaker 'inferior' peoples.[93] B.W. Ike in his paper *Apologetics of War*[94] quotes General von Hegel and Darwin being used to justify war as a legitimate method of resolving disputes:

> War is a biological necessity of the first importance, a regulative instrument in the life of mankind which cannot be dispensed with, since without it an unhealthy development will follow ... war is not only a biological necessity, it is also in some certain cases a moral obligation, and, as such, an indispensable factor of civilisation. The desire for peace has rendered most civilised nations anaemic, and marks a decay of spirit and political courage...[95]

Nicolai rejected this view outright and hoped that war would be abolished because *it had no biological value*. Like Richet, he saw the First World War as a process where selection had become negative. The brave, young, strong men were dying on the battlefields and the 'sickly and idiotic' were surviving at home. War could only act as a selective force if it was waged as a war of extermination of the enemy and this would only be possible if the enemy were not looked upon as human beings. He hoped that an enemy could never be dehumanised to the extent that would allow their extermination.[96] On the causes of war between nations, Nicolai thought that a 'tribal instinct' played an important part in the process. This tribal instict had compelled men to band together, because they were social beings, and as a result speech had developed, bonding each tribe more closely together. The families which were formed due to this process developed a 'racial instinct'. Tribal and racial instincts and love of one's native soil were, Nicolai thought, the roots of patriotism. Patriotism was one of the main factors in fuelling a war mentality:

> ... without patriotism war would be inconceivable today ... therefore the way small groups of individuals cling together, thereby impeding the solidarity of mankind, ought to be blamed, not praised.[97]

Unable to get a post in Germany after the war (because of his pacifist activities between 1914 and 1918 and his role in working for the peace and democratic organisations founded in Germany after the First World War) Nicolai was forced into exile in South America. He was appointed to several prestigious posts at universities in this continent, becoming a respected and influential teacher and thinker. Nicolai remained in South America where he died in 1964, mostly ignored by his fellow countrymen.

Dr Wilfred Trotter (1872–1939): The Herd Instinct

Writing in 1916 Wilfred Trotter, who, like Nicolai, was an eminent surgeon of his day, identified a cause of war different from Nicolai's tribal instinct. Trotter had become interested in the psychology of the time and had met Freud at a psycholanalytic congress in Vienna in 1908.[98] In *Instincts of the Herd in Peace and War*[99] Trotter attempted to show why it was that the behaviour of some groups of animals could not be explained using the three primitive instinctive categories of self-preservation, nutrition and sex. He identified a fourth instinct – gregariousness.[100] This manifested itself in a 'herd instinct'. Trotter suggested that herd traditions and herd thoughts were superior in their influence to individual reason, and he blamed the struggle between the two for conflicts not caused by physical environmental influences. Three types of development in herd life were postulated: that of animals who united for aggression as do wolves (he likened the

Germans to this category); that of the species like sheep, whose cohesion gives protection; and finally the highest degree of gregariousness, which he termed the socialised type, like the bee and the ant (in this class he put the English and Americans). As Holdstock points out:

> Instincts in the sense in which Trotter uses the term are fixed biological characters. Differences in national behaviour cannot, therefore, be instinctive in this way, and the sheep, the bees and the wolves no more than analogies. The comparison also neglects the essential difference between human aggression which is intra-specific, and that of the carnivore, which is a strategy for obtaining food.[101]

One of the characteristics of a herd member was not to be conspicuous; for example, to imitate the same dress, attitudes and nationalistic fervour as the other group members. Gregariousness can lead to unquestioning acceptance of herd dogma, and this works against individual thinking and expression and open-mindedness . . . which are necessary for progress.

Dr Sigmund Freud (1856–1939): The Primitive Instincts

Prompted by the outbreak of the First World War, Sigmund Freud in *Thoughts for the Times on War and Death*[102] discussed why it was that individuals were prepared to go to war, and the disillusionment that war had evoked amongst non-combatants. Society, Freud thought, had told itself that, although conflict between nations was in some cases inevitable, if it did occur then people 'expected the developed, civilised, dominating white races to have devloped better ways (other than war) of settling misunderstanding and conflicts of interests, such as international arbitration and through an international police force'.[103] Thus, when it began, the First World War with all its horrors brought disillusionment, disregarding as it did all International Law and moral standards which were promoted by the states themselves in peacetime. Freud identified two factors which aroused the sense of disillusionment in people:

1. Low morality shown externally by states which in their internal relations pose as the guardians of moral standards.
2. Brutality shown by individuals who, as participants in the 'highest

human civilisation', one would not have thought capable of such behaviour.

In peacetime, civilised society demands good behaviour. In exerting this pressure the primitive instinctual dispositions (primal needs) are suppressed and the influence of the cultural history of our ancestors is ignored. As a result there is an increasing tension and living with this 'hypocrisy' means that people are not living with the 'psychological truth'.[104]

In times of conflict, the primal needs which require satisfaction, by instinctual impulses, manifest themselves in an evil fashion. War enables the collective individuals to withdraw from *the constant pressure of civilisation* to grant temporary satisfaction to the instincts which they have been holding in check. Thus both state and individuals commit acts of brutality which should not be possible in such developed society.

Medical psychologist John MacCurdy in 1918 felt that Freud and Trotter were probably the only two psychologists, at the time of the First World War, who had initiated hypotheses that were not essentially tautological. He summarised what suggestions could be made as to the psychology of war:

> It is the natural outcome of fundamental human tendencies. Man by his gregarious nature is doomed to split up into groups, and these groups behave biologically as if they were separate species struggling for existence. Thanks to his herd instinct, which makes man accept the opinions of those immediately around him – herd or 'mob' suggestions – only that seems to be right which is done by the group, and an abnormal suspicion of the acts of other groups develops. Thus a state of antagonism develops which is much augmented by the aggressive tendency latent in human gregariousness. The antagonism is accumulative, so that sooner or later a state of extreme tension is reached. At this point, when action of some sort seems imperative, the primitive, unconscious instincts of man assert themselves (as they constantly tend to do), and the herd, finding in this a ready weapon, relaxes its ban, making of blood lust a virtue. Suddenly the individualistic and social tendencies find themselves working hand in hand . . . and

war with its tremendous energy is unleashed. The behaviour of both the mass and the individual then demonstrates that the herd is playing the role of a species struggling for existence.[105]

NOVEMBER 1918: WAR ENDS

As has been seen the great hopes of internationalism and world peace, actively promoted by the medical peace movement and others, had been dashed with the outbreak of hostilities in 1914. The Great War was fought at a cost of ten million lives with destruction on a scale not seen before, leaving the belligerents economically ruined. Jean de Bloch's prediction as to the future of war had come true; the powers of destruction were gaining on the powers of creation.[106] At its end there was great hope that the suffering it had brought would lead to a more secure and peaceful world. Sadly, as history records, and the following pages show, these dreams and aspirations were not to be. Despite the considerable efforts of all those working within the peace movement, the sad cycle of confrontation and conflict was to be repeated and the world again subjected to the full force of man's destructive capabilities.

PART THREE: 1919–45

Before detailing the medical profession's peace campaigns, it is useful to provide a summary of the political background of Europe between the wars.

RISE OF FASCISM

On 28 June 1919, the Treaty of Versailles was signed between France, the United States and Great Britain and the defeated German Empire. The terms of the treaty were harsh: Germany lost 13 per cent of her territory and 10 per cent of her population; colonies were taken away to be administered by the victorious allies; and the German army was reduced to 100,000 men. (Under the Treaty the German armed forces would not be allowed to possess tanks, heavy artillery, or a military air force and its navy would not be permitted to form a submarine force.) The Allies identified the arms race as one of the major causes of the war and singled out German militarism in particular. There was no mention of war reparations in the Treaty itself, but the principle was accepted in Article 231, the 'war guilt clause'.[1] Under this clause, the defeated powers accepted 'the responsibility of Germany and her allies for causing all the loss and damage to which Allied and Associated Governments and their nationals have been subjected as a consequence of the war imposed upon them by the aggression of Germany and her allies'. This clause justified the imposition of reparations, but no fixed sum was written into the Treaty because the Allies could not agree on one. Germany was required to hand over immediately £1,000 million to meet the cost of occupation and essential food imports. These conditions imposed on Germany were to be used in the 1920s to telling effect in German propaganda, with the emergence of Adolf Hitler and Fascism.

In Italy, Benito Mussolini (who had split with the Italian Socialist

Party in 1915 because he supported the entry of Italy into the First World War) formed the *Fascio di Combattimento* in 1919. In 1922 Mussolini sent 30,000 blackshirts to Rome and, overawed by this show of strength, the King gave him dictatorial powers for one year.[2] Within that year the Fascists consolidated their position, and Italy was soon to become a one-party state.

The rise to power of Hitler and the Nazi Party in Germany was aided by the memory and the economic consequences of the humiliating terms of the Treaty of Versailles, particularly the 'war guilt' clause it contained. Hitler had long been a right-wing activist and it was in 1923, whilst serving a year-long gaol sentence for his part in the failed Munich *putsch*, that he wrote *Mein Kampf*. By January 1933 Hitler's Nazis were the largest political force in Germany and he was appointed Chancellor of the Reichstag. In February of that year the Reichstag mysteriously caught fire, just before elections were due to be held in March, and suspicion as to the cause lay with Nazi Party members. Goering, however, quickly denounced the incident as a communist plot and used it as an excuse to arrest the communist leaders.

Violence was commonplace at this time with gangs of Nazis and communists engaged in street fighting. After the elections, Hitler declared the communist party illegal and forbade their elected representatives to take up their parliamentary responsibilities. By July 1933 Hitler had managed to suppress all other parties (mostly through terror tactics) and was in firm control of all government departments. He was able to announce that: 'There is only one political party in Germany — the Nationalist Socialist Workers Party'.[3] The party members' battle cry — *Ein Volk, Ein Reich, Ein Führer* — and their nationalistic, anti-semitic and anti-communist sentiments were given full lease.

With military and economic help from Hitler and Mussolini, the Spanish Civil War (1936–39) ended with the defeat of the republican forces, and General Franco set up Europe's third Fascist state. Although Spain managed to remain neutral during the Second World War, the civil war had provided a valuable training ground for German air forces and demonstrated the effectiveness of the aerial bombing strategies developed by Goering.

S.J. Woolf writes that Fascism, as an effective movement, was born out of fear.[4] In 1917 the Russian Revolution had broken out, and from 1917 to 1923 the Bolsheviks were preaching not socialism in one country, but world revolution. The force and dynamism of Fascism sprang from the fear of a new, and this time a 'proletarian', revolution. Woolf continues:

> European fascism, then, is the political response of the European bourgeoisie to the economic recession after 1918 – or rather more directly, to the political fear caused by that recession. Before all else, it was anti-communist.[5]

LEAGUE OF NATIONS

The League was established on 1 January 1920 with the Treaty of Versailles. On the surface its aims were simple. It existed to promote peace, and would do so through disarmament and negotiation. The powers were to work together to stop aggression and to try to build a world in which aggression became less likely. The most difficult question was whether a will to peace could be created, through the conduit of the League, in the peoples and governments of the world.[6] Its value received a major setback when Congress in the United States withdrew its support and President Wilson who had campaigned vigorously for the idea was voted out of office.

With the advent of the League, many of the pre-war peace movement's aspirations had been realised. Beales writes:

> There were to be no more crusades for arbitration treaties, no more frenzied petitions for the codification of International Law. Within the framework of the League, Governments had now taken up officially the work of preserving peace by co-operation.[7]

Membership of the League rose to some 60 states who agreed to the purpose of the League 'to prevent future wars by establishing relations on the basis of justice, honour and to promote co-operation, material and intellectual, between the nations of the world'. Although the League had some successes in managing conflict (such as the invasion of Albania by Yugoslavia in 1921, and in 1925 when Bulgaria invaded Greece), in major strategic clashes of interest the League proved ineffectual. This was certainly the case when dealing with totalitarian powers, for example when Mussolini invaded Abyssinia (1935) and Japan did likewise in Manchuria (1931) – they simply withdrew from the League. In 1932 the League tackled the question of disarmament at the Disarmament Conference, but in 1935 these ongoing talks broke down. Final blows to any authority and prestige it may have had came when Germany annexed Austria and Czechoslovakia, and the League offered no resistance. During the Second World War the technical side of the League's work (e.g. economic and health sections) continued to some degree from offices in New York. Later, the United Nations Organisation was to take over the material assets of the League and also some of its political and technical functions.

THE 'TRIPLE CRISIS' OF 1936

Martin Ceadel considers three main events in 1936 together constituted the major watershed of the decade.[8] These were the remilitarisation of the Rhineland in March, the final defeat of Abyssinia in May, and the civil war which broke out in Spain in July. The crises sparked off a debate between those who favoured a policy of containment and those who favoured accommodation. Containment was favoured by the League of Nations Union and the New Commonwealth Society and those who supported collective security. The problem with this was that containment was the policy blamed for the First World War. Since it was widely believed arms races caused wars – the concept of deterrence being little understood – those advocating rearmament were accused of fatalistically accepting the inevitability of war. Accommodation was more obviously a peace policy. It took two forms: for a hard core, pacifism; for the majority, appeasement.[9] Pacifists thought that total disarmament would morally deter aggressors or, if this failed, an invading army would be disabled by Gandhian non-violence. The Peace Pledge Union (PPU), after 1937, supported appeasement, a policy also supported by non-pacifists. Any hope of accommodating Germany was finally destroyed when Hitler invaded Czechoslovakia in March 1939.

THE PEACE MOVEMENT AFTER THE FIRST WORLD WAR

Women's International League for Peace and Freedom

Before leaving their Hague Conference in 1915 the women delegates had agreed to meet again after the war had ended. In 1919 one hundred and fifty assembled at Zurich at the same time that the 'peacemakers' were meeting at Versailles. The International Committee of Women for Permanent Peace (ICWPP) was renamed the Women's International League for Peace and Freedom (WILPF), and this latter group was quick to criticise the Treaty of Versailles for its harsh terms and the continuing food blockade. On this last issue Aletta Jacobs, Alice Hamilton and a few others undertook a study tour of Germany to see for themselves the effect that the food shortage, as a result of the Allied blockage, was having on the population, particularly the children. After the tour Jacobs immediately began to agitate for the provision of relief to the German people. She also discovered that there were almost half a million 'forgotten' German and other prisoners of war being held captive in Siberia, and initiated an action committee to promote their repatriation. This work was eventually taken over by the ICRC and the League of Nations, particularly through the efforts of Fridjof Nansen.

War Resisters International

After the war the conscientious objection movement re-organised as the No More War Movement, founded in February 1921. Representatives of war objector groups from four European countries met later in 1921, in Holland, and formed Paco (Esperanto for peace). By the end of 1922 members of Paco started using the term 'war resistance' and in 1923 Paco changed its name to War Resisters International (WRI), with headquarters in Hoddesdon, England. At its first international conference in 1925 the declaration of WRI was confirmed:

> **War is a crime against humanity. I, therefore, am determined not to support any kind of war and to strive for the removal of all causes of war.**[10]

WRI got much of its inspiration from the non-violent techniques which Gandhi had developed in India's struggle for independence. At the 1934 WRI conference held in England, Bart de Ligt put forward his Plan of Campaign against All War and All Preparation for War.[11] Some modern theoreticians and practitioners of direct non-violent action still consider de Ligt's plan 'the most systematic plan of a non-violent struggle against militarism available'.[12] As part of his plan he proposed the individual action of the medical man in peacetime in two parts:

1. *Indirect abstentionist methods* (i.e. a refusal to prepare a war-like mentality): by revealing the unconscious and subconscious tendencies which make for war, and the retrogressive character of military discipline, and by showing that modern war is an odious crime against life, the physical, the moral and mental health of man as well as against his aesthetic sense (millions dead, mutilated, unbalanced, sexual illnesses, consequences of undernourishment, TB, rachitis, etc.).
2. *Indirect constructive methods* (i.e. by preparing a humanitarian and international mentality):
    a. by analysing the pathological phenomena of society with a view to individual and social self-cure and the establishment of moral hygiene;
    b. by demonstrating the possibilities of canalising and sublimating the instincts and passions which formerly found their outward expression in war.

With the foundation of WRI an international pacifist organisation of wider scope than any before the First World War was initiated. This was a result of the commitment of dedicated conscientious objectors and pacifist activists during that war.

During the 1930s members of the medical profession also began to organise themselves and started campaigning publicly on subjects of war and peace. Their peace work complemented that of the peace movement as a whole, but also introduced particular areas of knowledge and expertise into the debate.

European Medical Peace Groups in the 1930s

Dutch Committee for the Prophylaxis of War: Netherlands

In 1930 a group of physicians and psychologists in the Netherlands attempted to bring the peace/war issue to the attention of the medical profession and a wider public. They persuaded the Netherlands Medical Association to establish the 'Dutch Committee for the Prophylaxis of War'. The term 'prophylaxis' was chosen deliberately to give it a medical flavour. In October 1935 they published a *Letter to the Statesmen* which was signed by 340 physicians, psychiatrists and psychologists from 28 countries and sent to the world's 'leading statesmen'. It started:

> We psychiatrists, whose duty it is to investigate the normal and

diseased mind, and to serve mankind with our knowledge, feel impelled to address a serious word to you in our quality as physicians. As in all things human, psychological factors play a very important part in the complicated problem of war... If war is to be prevented the nations and their leaders must understand their own attitudes towards war.[13]

The letter went on to challenge some leaders' opinions that war was a glorious affair, was the 'supreme court of appeal' and that war was the 'necessary outcome of Darwin's theory'. Ike[14] reports that the letter was well publicised and caught world-wide publicity. The other main achievement of this committee was the publication of *Medical Opinions on War*[15] which was a compilation of articles on the psychiatric and medical-psychological aspects of war. It is worth noting some of the issues raised by the authors since they will reappear in later assessments on these topics.

Dr Robert Thompson, in discussing a possible mediatory role for physicians, said:

> In the solution of a difficult issue between individuals or between nations... when each side appears to have a good case... the role of the mediator is of great importance. The mediator, however, must be of such standing as to command the respect of both sides and he should feel equal to the task before undertaking it, or the solution may be made worse. Also there is an optimum time to intervene. Too early intervention will be resented as undue interference, while if delayed too long tempers may have become too frayed to be assuaged.[16]

Macdonald Ladell, also writing in *Medical Opinions on War,* advocated that games for children of killing and wounding should be forbidden. War toys should not be sold and he even went as far as to suggest that children should watch 'the killing of some harmless animal... made deliberately painful and repulsive... to educate the child to the reality of death'. He also thought that war could be made unthinkable by divesting it of all the glamour and prestige which had collected around it, and the first step would be to get rid of all the verbal camouflage. What we mean now when we speak of war is organised mass murder (omnicide in today's terms) and we should say so. Men use words to make what they are doing seem less ghastly: for example, the pilots' saying of aircraft 'dropping eggs', not bombs, and so on. Modern military language has also developed the same tricks, such as 'collateral damage' for civilian deaths and casualties, 'take out' for kill, and so on. Macdonald articulated what psychologists now call 'mirror imaging':

> ... people picture their neighbours across the frontier as ready to let loose the horrors [of war] upon them, and they see their neighbours not as kindly, friendly human beings like themselves but as devils thirsting for their destruction.[17]

Also writing in *Medical Opinions on War*, Leonard Browne restated the view that peace is not merely the absence of war (negative peace), whether military or economic, but must be a harmony of trust and cooperation between nations (positive peace). Talking of the image that the peacemaker has, he noted that for many people war-making appears more glorious than peacemaking. The warrior always appears more virile and more positive than the peacemaker. He thought it necessary for the cause of peace to be presented positively so that it may:

> ... arouse the energies and enthusiasm of the more intelligent people, who after all are the decisive factor in an effort of this kind... The arousing of feeling must be followed by practical action as a constructive plan, otherwise the desire for peace 'peters out'.[18]

The object of the collection of articles was, as Dr Roorda wrote in the preface, 'to enlarge the self knowledge of common citizens and politicians'. They did not pretend to present any scientific discoveries, but to sound the voice of medical common sense. This tradition of public education is continued by the medical peace groups of today.

MEDICAL PEACE CAMPAIGN: GREAT BRITAIN

1936 saw Europe in the grip of the 'triple crisis'. In August of that year a letter was published in *The Lancet*, headed 'The Medical Peace Campaign' (MPC).[19] This called on doctors who supported the four points of the International Peace Campaign (IPC) to communicate with the secretary of the MPC, so that members of the medical profession attending the imminent Peace Congress in Brussels could feel that they had the 'support of a substantial number of colleagues'. The four points in question were:

1. Recognition of the sanctity of treaty obligations.
2. Reduction and limitation of armaments by international agreement, and the suppression of profit from the manufacture and trade in arms.
3. Strengthening the League of Nations for the prevention and stopping of war by the organisation of collective security and mutual assistance.
4. Establishment within the framework of the League of Nations of effective machinery for remedying international conditions which might lead to war.

At the IPC Congress (1936), the Medical and Psychological Sub-Commission passed several resolutions, the first of which stated:

> Owing to its special position, its special knowledge of health and disease, and its great influence on public opinion, the medical profession has a special duty to work actively for peace.[20]

Many of the members of MPC belonged to a group known as Psychologists for Peace, which had been formed several years earlier, influenced by correspondence between Freud and Einstein on the causes of war and hopes for peace.[21] Einstein had initiated this exchange, at the suggestion of the International Institute of Intellectual Co-operation based in Paris, and asked Freud various questions relating to man's behaviour and attitude towards war.[22] Freud said that he had no straightforward answers but thought that humanity was innately aggressive and linked this aggressiveness to his own theory of the 'death instinct'. Einstein thought our aggression could not be eliminated so our hope came from the strengthening of its opposing tendency – the development of emotional bonds between men, enhanced by common interests and by identification.[23] As in 1915, Freud wrote of the influence of the process of civilisation on delaying war impulses which were inherent in society.

Like the Dutch Committee the MPC's main achievement, other than getting the issues discussed in a wider arena within the medical profession and the population as a whole, was the publication of a book. *The Doctor's View on War*[24] was published in 1938 and in its foreward Professor John Ryle voiced a dream:

> By withholding service from the armed forces before and during war, by declining to examine and innoculate recruits, by refusing sanitary advice and the training and command of ambulances, clearing stations, medical transports, and hospitals, the doctors could so cripple the efficiency of the staff and aggravate the difficulties of the campaign and so damage the morale of the troops that war would become almost unthinkable ... in such a refusal of service ... there would be no inhumanity comparable with the inhumanity which medicine at present sanctions and prolongs [vis-à-vis war]. But let the dream pass and fantasy make room for facts.

In Chapter 9 of the book some concern is expressed that the state may involve doctors in a war or war situation through state organisation that conflicts with the doctor's moral position.[25] The traditional independence of the medical profession was seen as being undermined. With the emergence of a more strident nationalism, which seemed to deny any universal and international truth and with its conception of war as a totalitarian one, it was felt that the state would insist that doctors made a choice, simply, 'for us or against us'. The MPC felt that as doctors they had good reason to object to the principle of intensified nationalism and to its application, not only in Hitler's Germany, but also possibly in Great Britain at some future date.

Before the Second World War there was debate on whether doctors should become involved as volunteer 'national emergency' medical officers. What, it was asked, is a national emergency? The official definition was given as 'when the territorial forces are mobilized'. The concern expressed was that if, for example, a national emergency was declared in the event of a miners' strike – with which a good many doctors may have sympathy – with whom should their obligations lie? What would a doctor's duty be if a war arose, the reasons for which they did not agree with? There were overt threats made to doctors who did not reply to a circular sent to them requesting them to register as 'volunteers'. Not only were they thought to be upatriotic, but one letter received by a general practitioner, who did not register, said:

... those doctors who have been given the chance of home service [now] will be the last to be called upon, should an emergency arise, for active service abroad. Those doctors who have not returned their forms will probably not receive the same consideration.[26]

In the conclusion of *The Doctor's View on War* a call was made for an international conference of medical societies. It was hoped that, for the sake of humanity, a call from the conference would be made for a system of collective security to be established at an international level ... or a reversion to barbarism was inevitable. In a review of the book *The Lancet* commented:

> We fear that conflicting loyalties would make it almost impossible for such a gathering [the proposed conference] to reach substantial agreement.[27]

A few weeks after the letter regarding the MPC which had been published in *The Lancet* on 22 August 1936, Dr D. A. Crow, speaking at the annual meeting of the Brighton Division of the British Medical Association, referring to the profession's duty in helping to prevent war, said:

> If war breaks out, the medical profession will throw all its weight of unselfish effort into the turmoil, and in the end will have done nothing but help, as far as is possible, to clear up the mess. I want to know why a great and powerful profession, such as our own, should not make some vivid gesture toward minimizing the risk of such a mess occurring at all.[28]

Because the *British Medical Journal* refused to print his speech in full, Dr Crow published it himself in the form of a pamphlet entitled *The British Medical Association versus The British Warfare Association*.[29] The article in *Peace News* applauds the fact that here is a doctor who is not one of the usual members of a 'medical profession inclined to be reactionary in its political outlook', and ends by quoting the pamphlet's conclusion:

> It is the old, old conflict between those who would create and those who would destroy, and our profession is a poor concern if

all we do is to pick up the bits and pieces of a shattered world, knowing all the time that we should have been in the very forefront of its creative force.

Civil Defence (CD) was a major campaigning issue for the MPC. An editorial 'Preparation for Air-Raids'[30] endorsed a request to the British Medical Association (BMA) to organise a committee of enquiry into the effects of an attack by hostile aircraft on the city of London. The editorial noted that:

1. The public did not understand the probable effects of attacks on great cities from the air
2. The public relied unduly on such armour as the gas mask and the gas-proof room (see below).
3. The government, seeking above all things the preservation of order during an emergency, was not being frank about the inadequacy of the provision it could make in advance.

These points have a familiar ring to critics of present-day CD planning. In 1937 the Cambridge Scientists Anti-War Group in its publication *Protection of the Public from Aerial Attack*[31] gave a detailed critique of Home Office plans for 'gas-proof rooms' to be constructed, by civilians, as protection against air bombardment by poison gas. It also examined the efficacy of gas masks and protection against incendiary bombs and high explosives. *The Lancet* hoped that the scientific committee of enquiry could do something effective also in the *prevention of war*, noting that others looked upon it merely as a means of attempting to *prevent unnecessary casualties* once war had broken out. Finally, the article said that members of the medical profession had a duty towards all mankind and, as such, owed no allegiance to governments or government departments.

Not all comment in *The Lancet* was favourable towards the MPC. In 'Grains and Scruples',[32] the columnist wrote expressing the opinion that the intrusion of amateurs, like MPC, into this expert field of war and its causes, could even make war more likely, and could not engender peace. To psychologists dogmatising about international affairs he said:

> Psychotherapeutic techniques, which have not as yet been uniformly successful in individual disorders, should be used spar-

ingly in international affairs – and when used it should be limited in its application to the psychotherapist's own countrymen... Nothing makes me more warlike than the pronouncements of some psychologists on peace.

The MPC struggled on in its opposition to war and in May 1939, four months before the outbreak of the Second World War, Professor John Ryle, then its president, made a plea for Great Britain, France and Russia to stand united to resist all further aggression by military force. He reminded colleagues that, as members of the most international and humane of all professions, they could still play a vital role in influencing public opinion on behalf of peace. But war broke out and the activities of the MPC ceased.

The White Sickness

Peace News of 27 February 1937 reports an item of some interest to doctors. Under the heading 'Karel Capek's New Peace Play'[33] a report is given of the production of a play by the famous Czech dramatist and pacifist, Karel Capek, called *The White Sickness*. *Peace News* reports that the hero was a doctor who had discovered a cure for an imaginary disease which the author called 'the white sickness'. The doctor, a fervent pacifist, refused to treat an arms manufacturer who had this disease unless he promised to give up his factory. In the meantime, the dictator of his country attacks a weak neighbouring state without warning. The dictator himself is stricken with the mysterious disease and eventually dies at the same time as the pacifist doctor.

Help with the moral dilemmas facing doctors on whether or not to become involved with their country's war preparations came from Dick Sheppard and the PPU.

Advice to Doctors from Dick Sheppard

In October 1934 Canon 'Dick' Sheppard appealed to men to pledge themselves against war by sending him a postcard saying that they bound themselves by the pledge:

> *I renounce war and never again will I support or sanction another, and I will do all in my power to persuade others to do the same.*

Out of this was born the Peace Pledge Union which by October 1936 had 100,000 members.[34] Physicians wanted to know from him – 'Does this rule out the Royal Army Medical Corps (RAMC) as well as the combat units?' In reply Sheppard advised:

> The pledge does not mean that we refuse to succour the wounded. To do so is an elementary Christian duty. But here the doctor who is a pacifist finds himself in a dilemma. If he accepts a commission in the RAMC he becomes subject to military discipline, and must obey the orders of the Army medical authority... during the Great War 82 per cent of the wounded in the British Forces were utimately returned to duty, 64 per cent of them to the front line. A doctor who contributed to such a result would undoubtedly be helping to wage, and to probably prolong, the war in which he was serving as a medical officer.[35]

Sheppard suggests that the pacifist doctor would be justifed in staying at home caring for the civilians and war-related diseases, such as the medical effects of poor nutrition and the corresponding increase in diseases such as gonorrhea, syphilis and TB, associated with war and large armies. But if this action also meant that the time came when men remained unattended in war zones, and the most effective remedy would be for him to go to the front, then the doctor should reconsider his position because 'he is vowed to the healing of men – and to tend to those who need his care is his first duty. In these circumstances, however, it would probably be easy for him to retain his civilian status. *If any large number of doctors insisted on doing so, the authorities would have no option but to yield.*'

No account of physicians' involvement in peace issues for the period leading up to the outbreak of the Second World War would be complete without mention of the great Italian doctor and educationalist, Maria Montessori.

DR MARIA MONTESSORI: EDUCATOR FOR PEACE

Maria Montessori (1870–1952) was neither a political activist nor a feminist. After first studying engineering, she entered the University of Rome from where she graduated in 1896, with the first MD awarded to a woman in Italy.[36] She developed an interest in the education of mentally deficient children, and travelled to London and Paris to study the techniques of Jean Itard and Edouard Seguin in particular. The results of her work with these children were dramatic and her success made her wonder why the same principles could not be applied for the benefit of 'normal' children. Her opportunity came in 1906 when the city of Rome invited Montessori to provide a teaching facility for children living in a progressive housing project which they were developing. *Casa dei bambini* had been set up in the tenement blocks and it was with the children attending these nursery schools that she applied the key elements of the teaching system she had developed with her mentally retarded children at the university clinic. Put very simply these were: self-education; an appeal to the intellect – she felt that the ultimate reference is to the sense of touch, which is regarded as fundamental and primordial;[37] self-restraint on behalf of the teachers and parents so as not to impose their personalities on the children; non-competitive, that is, no prizes or marks but a fostering of the co-operative spirit. Once again she achieved remarkable results and 'Montessori' schools became established all over the world.

In 1932 Montessori gave her first lecture on the theme of education for peace at the International Bureau of Education. 'War is like plague,' she said, 'and it leaves us bewildered. But just as a new physical constitution was needed to defeat plague, so we need a new spiritual constitution to help us put an end to war.'[38] The 'spiritual' side of a child's development must not be ignored. It was important that schools were not regarded as the breeding ground for war, in that instead of developing a child's sociability, in many cases they discouraged it.[39] In 1934 she left Italy (feeling that Mussolini's Fascist regime was seeking to exploit her international reputation), going first to Spain and finally settling in the Netherlands. It was during the last two decades of her life that she spoke out most strongly for peace. Two of the nine international Montessori congresses she organised were devoted to peace and education (at Copenhagen in 1937, and San Remo, Italy, 1949).[40] Whilst in Copenhagen she met Bart de Ligt, the famous Dutch exponent of non-violence, a 'revolutionary' pacifist and member of WRI, which was also holding a conference in that city. De Ligt reported that Montessori:

> was much concerned with the fact that the modern military state

was assailing more and more the divine possibilities inherent in the child, this 'new world citizen without any rights'.[41]

Montessori also sent a written message to the International Congress against War and Militarism held in Paris, 1–5 August 1937, in which she said:

> A war would be such an undoubted danger for mankind that it is the duty of every one of us to act with energy to prevent its coming. The method which you have chosen is the most direct, and if adopted would bring an end to all danger of future war.

and

> ... If at some time the Child were to receive proper consideration and his immense possibilities were to be developed, then a Man might arise for whom there would be no need of encouragement to disarmament and resistance to war because his nature would be such that he could not endure the state of degradation and of extreme moral corruption which makes possible any participation in war.[42]

At the outbreak of the Second World War Maria Montessori was teaching in India, and, being an Italian national, was interned. The course of the war strengthened her belief that a radical reform of the entire educational system was necessary. She saw peace positively, not being just the absence of war, and firmly believed that education should play a vital role so that 'it no longer stifles the normal development of individuals but rather fosters the spiritual liberation of humanity'.[43]

Montessori died in 1952 after a life dedicated to children and a complete trust for the future in children, given the right care, nurture and opportunities. She was nominated for the Nobel Peace Prize in 1949, 1950 and 1951.

ROLE OF THE RED CROSS QUESTIONED

Before closing this section reference should be made to the activities of the Red Cross at this time. It should be remembered that, from the outset, the organisation was conceived to relieve victims but not to prevent war. Of course, the Red Cross is not indifferent to the problem of war in general – it feels that it has contributed greatly to the spirit of peace engendered by its traditional humanitarian work. The effectiveness of this work depends on respect for its neutrality, respect for its symbol on the battlefield and on non-interference (politically).[44]

But in 1938 the role of the Red Cross came under discussion. A *Lancet* editorial headed 'The Red Cross: An End or Beginning?' listed the abuses of the Red Cross symbol in the Abyssinian/Italian conflict and the Spanish Civil War and expressed the opinion that in modern totalitarian war the distinction between medical and other branches of the fighting services was lessened.[45] The medical profession and such organisations as the Red Cross societies and ambulance associations came under the direction of the military who (in the editor's opinion), in time of war, controlled the state. The 'red cross' was no longer a symbol of neutrality and no longer a symbol of service that recognised no difference between men of differing beliefs and races. A revival of its respect would be aided with the founding of a definite movement – with members of medical and allied professions in all countries – to ensure that the principles of mutual aid would be applied to mankind. A change of heart was required. To achieve a revival of the founding ideas of the Red Cross and universal mutual aid, miracles would have to be achieved by 'co-operation and self-denial'. The editorial summed up:

> For in the circumstances of today it is all too evident that nearly all of us are English or German or Japanese or communists or property owners before we are doctors and scientists.[46]

THE SECOND WORLD WAR (1939–45)

The advent of the Second World War in September 1939 confronted pacifists with the old dilemma – whether to take part or not. Many who had signed Sheppard's Peace Pledge joined up, seeing in Hitler and Nazism an evil that required forceful opposition – it was a 'just war'. Boards were set up by the government to consider requests for exemption from military service from conscientious objectors (COs). These were pacifists from both secular and religious groups who had been active before the Second World War. Although COs did undergo some harassment because of their stand, it was not to the same extent as during the First World War. Some were imprisoned, particularly the 'absolutists' who refused to accept alternatives offered in the civilian sector, since they saw, even in this, help towards the state's war machine.

Some found other solutions after much soul-searching. One doctor writes:

> I was registered as a C.O. unconditionally and in a reserved job but I came to feel that it was wrong to be in safety and rely on the Merchant Navy to bring me food, so I joined the Merchant Navy, not very logical but in total war you either support the 'war effort' by taking alternative service – social work, fire service, land work etc., or you go to prison and inevitably are a drag on the community and so help the enemy. I cannot see a way around this moral dilemma...[47]

A Central Board for Conscientious Objection (CBCO) was set up in 1940 to lobby on behalf of COs and to support them by looking after their interests – so as to ensure no mistreatment was taking place in prisons. The pacifist response through the CBCO concentrated on the provision of legal advice to COs rather than direct war resistance of any kind. It was illegal in Britain to persuade people to avoid military service – activists so doing would be charged with conspiracy. In other countries no war resistance whatsoever was tolerated, and pacifists faced execution for their stand against war.

PART FOUR: 1946–90

PERIODS OF ACTIVITY IN THE PEACE MOVEMENT: A SUMMARY

A review of the literature reveals several typologies of activity in the peace movement between 1946 and 1990 and this section of the book will incorporate the following schemes, in which the medical peace movement was active. Young[1] identifies three significant waves of support after 1945, periods of *mass involvement* in the British peace movement:

1. 1945–49: on nuclear issues.
2. 1966–70: during the Vietnam War.
3. 1979–84: on nuclear issues.

Wittner[2] sees three international waves of *nuclear disarmament sentiment:*

1. 1945–49: from Hiroshima to the Soviet manufacture of an atomic bomb.
2. 1957–63: generated by the escalation of the nuclear arms race, atmospheric testing and proliferation.
3. 1979–83: another surge in the nuclear arms race symbolised by a breakdown of Soviet–American détente.

There are three main periods where *medical involvement in nuclear war concerns* is identified by Ike:[3]

1. Until mid-1960s when stress was laid on medical possibilities and obligations in the protection and treatment of war victims.
2. After mid-1960s when the truth about nuclear war had dawned on the medical world.
3. In 1980, the formation of International Physicians for the Preven-

tion of Nuclear War (IPPNW) saw the establishment of the idea of medical war prevention at international levels.

The apparent failure of the peace movement before 1939 to prevent the Second World War (coupled with the accusation of 'appeasement', the legacy of which still sticks) was probably one of the major reasons why it took so long for the movement to re-emerge as a relevant political factor after 1945.[4]

For the first few years after the Second World War the peace movement was led, and dominated, by communist organisations orchestrated from Moscow. The World Peace Council (WPC) had affiliates in many countries and these became increasingly anti-American. Wittner states that the self-serving nature of the communist-led peace campaign became increasingly evident after the beginning of the Korean War (1950–53). With increasing stridency the WPC denounced American 'war crimes' in Korea and nuclear disarmament continued to decline on its scale of priorities. In Eastern Europe also:

> ... as the WPC's 'peace struggle' became a euphemism for military preparations and Soviet foreign policy, it created widespread cynicism among the peoples of Eastern Europe. Here, as elsewhere, the communist led peace campaign did little more than discredit the cause that it claimed to represent.[5]

One of the first anti-war groups founded after the Second World War, in response to a perceived threat to world peace from the escalating confrontation between the communist and capitalist regimes around the world, was the Medical Associaton for the Prevention of War in the United Kingdom.

MEDICAL ASSOCIATION FOR THE PREVENTION OF WAR (MAPW)

A letter published in *The Lancet*, in January 1951, under the heading 'Prospect of War', began:

> There is an increasingly widespread assumption, both within the profession and elsewhere, that world war is inevitable. Concerned by this defeatist attitude we have met together to exchange ideas and now feel impelled to express ourselves publicly.[6]

The authors, most of whom had been active members of the MPC of the 1930s, went on to decry the assumpton that war with Stalin's expansionist Russia was inevitable and appealed to fellow doctors to join them:

> ... in the spirit of our chosen profession of healing, in doing all in their power to halt preparation for war and to bring about a new and determined approach to the peaceful settlement of disputes and to world disarmament.

The response in the letters columns of the following week was mixed. One writer commented that medicine and politics were 'together undergoing a shift to the left' and an 'already inglorious commensalism is being changed to a more violent parasitism'.[7]

'Bohemicus' compared the lack of freedom of expression and human rights in Czechoslovakia, Hungary and Poland with the necessity to defend our own freedoms by building up, and maintaining, adequate military strength.[8] Other letters were published in support of the signatories of 'Prospect of War'.

As a result of all this activity (and against the background of an increasingly acrimonious 'cold war'[9]) the Medical Association for the Prevention of War (MAPW) was inaugurated on 18 March 1951, with a membership of 130 doctors. The aims and objects of MAPW were to unite doctors in efforts to prevent war, and in particular:

1. To consider and formulate the ethical responsibilities of doctors in relation to war.
2. To study the causes and results of war.
3. To examine the psychological mechanisms by which people are conditioned to accept war as a necessity.
4. To oppose the use of medical science for any purpose other than the prevention and relief of suffering.
5. To urge that the energies and money spent in preparation for war against man be directed into the fight against disease and malnutrition.
6. To seek the co-operation of all doctors, in all countries, having the same aims.[10]

At the first MAPW meeting[11] views expressed included: a wish that doctors working on medicine in military research should resign from the profession; a concern about the relationship of the peace movement to the communists (this was to become an issue between the Labour Party and MAPW in 1953); the formation of an international unit for the care of war injured, owing allegiance to nobody; and to make use of international contacts within medicine to build up an international body, as proof against 'the present urge to war'. This latter objective was eventually achieved with the formation of IPPNW in 1980.

Contact was quickly made with other groups around the world such as the Union Nationale des Médicins pour la Paix which had been formed in France the previous year and was reputed to have a membership of 600. They had arranged a conference linking military spending on re-armament to serious deterioration in mental and physical health in France.[12] In 1952 another group linked with the medical profession was set up in France, the Comité de la Neutralité de la Médecine en Temps de Guerre.[13] The driving force behind this organisation was Professor Charles Richet (son of the famous French pacifist of the same name, and profession, already mentioned) who was professor in the Faculty of Medicine, University of Paris. Richet proposed that, in each country, a group of doctors and jurists who understood the conventions of the Red Cross should be set up in time of peace, so that they could be sent immediately to places where fighting breaks out. These groups would have a special international status, so that they would be accredited to all nations. If, as was possible, the war affected the whole world, the committees of doctors and jurists, with supranational status, would be morally neutral. They would be in the best position 'to enable our shattered civilisation to survive'. Not much is known about this Comité.[14]

In Denmark in 1952 the Danske Laegers Sammenslutning mod Krig (Danish Physicians against War) was created by a group of physicians including Sven Heinild, Hjalmar Helweg, H. C. A. Lassen and Ejnar Geert Jorgensen, which had 200–300 members. Klaus Arnung[15] makes the point, also applicable to other parts of the peace movement, how the arguments then for the involvement of physicians in peace matters resemble those of the 1980s and he quotes from their appeal for involvement:

> For every physician the question arises: is it at all possible in a

world – where 20–40 per cent of national budgets are used for weapons production and maintenance of the military apparatus because of reciprocal fear – also to secure sufficient resources for the struggle agianst disease; for the construction of new hospitals; for medical research; for improvement in housing conditions and general health standards. Reduction in arms spending is, in our opinion, a precondition for developing our profession for the benefit of humanity.

Their aims and objectives were very similar to those of MAPW. After three or four years the group gradually died out, mostly because its active members became involved in other concerns and also because of the heightening of the cold war.

In Belgium a 'Medical Group for the Maintenance of Peace' was set up;[16] in Italy doctors held a conference to discuss the impact of war preparation on health services; and in the US Quaker physicians had formed the Friends Medical Society which looked at peace issues. In the first years of its formation research was undertaken by MAPW members on chemical and biological warfare, the psychology of war and the ethical responsibilities of doctors during wartime.

DOCTORS CONFRONT GOVERNMENT WAR PLANNING

In the summer of 1951 a major row developed within the medical profession over a questionnaire, circulated to all doctors by the Central Medical War Committee (CMWC), asking for details likely to be useful in a 'fresh state of emergency' – widely regarded as a euphemism for nuclear war.[17] Many of the issues at stake, and opinions expressed, were similar to those used in the case of the 'volunteer emergency medical officers' in 1938. MAPW felt that the appearance and tone of the document at that time in the prevailing international situation (the Korean War had just started) actually contributed to the risk of war and reduced the possibility of conciliation... it ran the risk of creating an unwarranted impression of emergency at home and increasing suspicion abroad.[18] It was also suggested that the existence of the CMWC and the principles of the Hippocratic Oath were incompatible; that is, that doctors were being taught to endeavour always to preserve life, yet were now being asked to assist in a policy devoted to its mass destruction.[19] Dr Watney-Roe thought that the formation of a British Medical Association (BMA) Peace Committee, 'to consider ways and means of bringing home to everyone the folly, stupidity and wickedness of a drift towards war', would be appropriate.[20]

MAPW AND THE LABOUR PARTY: PROSCRIPTION

After considering the activities of MAPW, the National Executive Committee (NEC) of the Labour Party added the Association to its list of proscribed organisations on 25 February 1953. This meant that MAPW was ineligible for affiliation to the Labour Party (if it had wanted to do so), and that individual members were also ineligible for membership of the Labour Party. It was a time of in-fighting and division within the Party, when Stalinist factions were forming front groups to further their political aims, such as peace organisations, for example, Scientists for Peace and the British Peace Council. These were usually affiliated to the WPC which has already been mentioned. MAPW responded quickly, writing to the secretary of the Labour Party, Morgan Phillips, expressing their surprise at 'this astonishing and arbitrary decision'. The letter continues:

> MAPW is purely a professional body, with no connection with any political or other organisation. It is concerned solely with the ethical responsibilities of the profession and with the contribution which medical science can make to the lessening of inter-group tensions. The political independence of the Association could have been ascertained immediately by examination of its publications and of its record of activity, and from the personnel of its Officers and Executive Committee.
>
> We are not concerned with the harm which the action of your Committee will do to the Labour Party, but we are perturbed that it places one more barrier in the way of those who are trying to increase tolerance and understanding in the world.[21]

The problem appears to have arisen mainly over one event. In 1952 a member of MAPW's executive committee attended the Vienna Peace

Congress, which was sponsored by the WPC, and proscribed by the Labour Party NEC as being a 'bogus communist "peace" congress', under the domination of the communist WPC – which it undoubtedly was.[22] MAPW replied that a member of the executive committee attended as an *observer* only to report on the character and value of the Congress 'as is customary for an organisation to do when it does not desire to commit itself in any way to the policies of another organisation' and 'it has been our settled policy to appoint representatives only to such conferences as are *specifically medical or psychological in character*'.[23] Despite continued requests from MAPW to clear up this misunderstanding and requests to meet with representatives of the NEC, MAPW remained on the proscribed list until 1962. One cannot help feeling, from the evidence available, that the proscription was a result of general paranoia in the Labour Party due to the Stalinists' political assaults at that time. This 'smear' of communist influence was to be used 30 years later by members of the Conservative Party when peace movement activity peaked in the early 1980s.

One of the most influential voices within MAPW from its formation was that of Lionel Penrose, and he deserves a special mention.

MAPW AND PROFESSOR LIONEL PENROSE

Lionel Sharples Penrose (1898–1972) had also been active in the MPC before the Second World War. He came from a Quaker family with a strong anti-war tradition, had a brilliant career as a medical scientist (his work on genetics and mongolism was outstanding), and was deeply committed to the scientific study of war and its prevention.[24] Penrose favoured the interdisciplinary concept and this was a feature of the conferences he organised in which biologists, historians, economists, international lawyers and others participated. He undertook a major study on crowd behaviour using mainly mathematical methods, and formulated new insights on the mechanisms involved in group decision-making and the spread of ideas in populations.[25] He differed in this respect from Freud, Trotter and Nicolai who described and attempted to analyse the structure of the phenomena observed in terms of social or psychological concepts. He defended this 'numerical' approach in his book *On the Objective Study of Crowd Behaviour*[26] as follows:

The quantitative approach, though it may seem superficial in many respects, has the advantage over more traditional methods of social enquiry in that it lacks political or national bias. One of the causes of mental unrest in the world at the present time is the growing awareness among members of the human race of the vast extent of their own population. Thus is seems appropriate to pay attention to the reaction of crowds which are especially connected with or determined by the numbers of people they contain.

Penrose also made a mathematical analysis of voting procedure at the United Nations and formulated a fairer way of voting, which he regarded as an 'essential component in the mechanism of human civilisation'.[27]

MAPW continued to campaign against nuclear weapons and this was given more urgency with the explosion of the first hydrogen bomb in 1954.

DOCTORS PROTEST ABOUT THE H-BOMB

On 1 March 1954 the first hydrogen bomb was exploded by the US at Bikini Atoll in the Marshall Islands (the USSR did likewise in November 1955), an event which increased man's destructive capacity many times. The development of the hydrogen bomb was MAPW's main concern between 1953 and 1955[28] and an editorial on this topic in *The Lancet* stimulated a lively debate in the letters columns.[29] A month previously Professor A. Haddow, President of MAPW, in a letter to *The Times*[30] had issued a challenge to fellow scientists, as a direct result of the H-bomb explosion and the announcement that it was now possible to manufacture a 'dirty' cobalt bomb. Haddow stated in his letter:

> While the crisis is unlikely to be affected by the endeavour of any single individual today, such would not necessarily be so were the issues transferred under the aegis of the United Nations, to a *concilium* of world science, representing especially physics, chemistry, biology and medicine, representative also of their nationalities, yet supranational in outlook, of an authority trans-

cending that of the politician, and with an unimpeachable primary loyalty to humanity as a whole.

The scientists should meet to appraise the human situation created by the existence of the hydrogen bomb, and set themselves to devise policies to prevent its manufacture. Dr Alex Comfort wrote that the 'hydrogen bomb... is the mental patients' weapon *par excellence*. Atomic research in the US . . . has long since passed from the sphere of weapons research into that of abnormal psychology'.[31] Opposing these views Dr Stafford-Clark, in replying to Comfort's opinion that there was less menace from Russia than from the US, felt that the anti-bomb vocalists were 'playing into the hands of communist propaganda' and that for Britain to dissociate itself from its greatest ally (the US) 'would be to present the world with a free gift of tyranny'.[32] Other letters called for both East and West to halt aggressive propaganda; for Britain to become neutral (although some like Stafford-Clark felt that this would provide 'very favourable soil for malignant, ruthless and energetic efforts of communist infiltration'); and for effective international control of production and development of atomic weapons.

Concern about nuclear weapons and their effects was also voiced by Nobel Laureate Dr Albert Schweitzer, who began to speak out forcefully on these issues in the late 1950s particularly.

DR ALBERT SCHWEITZER: NOBEL PEACE PRIZE 1953

Albert Schweitzer (1875–1965) qualified in medicine at the age of 38 – he had orginally obtained a PhD in Theology from the University of Strasbourg in 1889 and had worked as a pastor. Influenced by the teachings of the Apostle Paul, his 'reverence for life' had made him a humanitarian, but not a politically active pacifist.[33] His calling led him to devote the rest of his life to working as a medical missionary in Africa. In recognition of his efforts at Lambarene leprosy hospital and other humanitarian medical work in Africa, Schweitzer was awarded the Nobel Peace Prize in 1953. He ended his Nobel Prize speech with Paul's words: 'If it be possible, as much as lieth with you, live peaceably with all men.'[34] Schweitzer became more outspoken in his anti-war beliefs after this time (partly due to the influence of his friends Albert

Einstein and Norman Cousins), and in 1958 he broadcast 'Three Appeals' from Oslo.[35] In these, he appealed

1. for an end to atmospheric testing,
2. for the nuclear powers to agree anti-proliferation measures, both vertical and horizontal;

and he supported

3. the formation of a nuclear weapons free zone, as suggested by Polish Foreign Minister Rapacki, in East and West Germany and Czechoslovakia.

Schweitzer remained involved in peace agitation and his last public effort, just before his death in 1965, was to call for a cease-fire in the Vietnam War.[36]

In 1957 two organisations were formed; whilst not purely medical groups, doctors made valuable contributions to them in the continuing debate about peace and world co-operation. Pugwash and Sane became 'active' in 1957, the beginning of a period, as we shall see later, of increasing anti-nuclear sentiment.

PUGWASH

In the International forum there was some activity with the formation of Pugwash in July 1957. This orgnisation was due mostly to the work of Bertrand Russell and Albert Einstein who had issued the Russell–Einstein Manifesto in July 1955, calling on scientists to assemble in a conference to discuss the means of averting the dangers resulting from the arms race and the development of the hydrogen bomb.[37] Scientists (including physicians) participated as individuals and not as the representative of any government or organisation. Rotblat says of the significance of this first conference:

> ... this was probably the first time that a truly international conference, organised by scientists, with participants from East and West, was convened not to discuss specific technical matters, but the social implications of scientific discovery.[38]

Professor Haddow, of MAPW, was an early participant in Pugwash. At the seventh conference a group looking at 'Preservation and Promotion of Health' noted that 'health sciences offer one of the most rewarding meeting grounds for international co-operation in science', and in 1980 the Pugwash Working Group issued a statement wishing it to be known that, in their view, medical disaster planning for a nuclear war was futile; that there is no possible effective medical response after a nuclear attack and that effective civil defence against nuclear attack is impossible.

SANE

In the United States the National Committee for a Sane Nuclear Policy (Sane) was also formed in 1957, partly in response to increasing fears over radioactive fallout from nuclear testing. Prominent in the activities of Sane were Dr Benjamin Spock, a famous pediatrician (one of Sane's newspaper adverts had featured Spock looking, with furrowed brow, at a child under the caption 'Dr Spock Is Worried'), and Dr Erich Fromm (1900–80), a leading psychoanalyst and social critic.[39] The name 'Sane' is reputed to have been derived from Fromm's book *The Sane Society*.[40] Fromm believed that since the First World War there had been an increasing indifference to life, an increasing brutalisation of man leading to a lessening of conscience, 'the essence of which is an inherent protest against the wanton destruction of life'.[41] This was weakening the basic form of ethical behaviour – the reverence for life, as Albert Schweitzer had formulated.

INCREASING NUCLEAR TENSIONS

Wittner characterised the period 1957 to 1963 as being marked by a powerful wave of anti-nuclear sentiment (of which Pugwash and Sane were a part), generated by the escalation of the nuclear arms race, proliferation, and worries over atmospheric fallout from the H-bomb tests.[42] The Russians launched Sputnik in 1957 and demonstrated successful tests of ICBMs, increasing US worries about their vulnerability to nuclear attack. In 1961 the tension in Europe heightened with the building of the Berlin Wall, and in 1962 the world came to the brink of nuclear war during the Cuba Crisis when the USSR attempted to deploy nuclear missiles in Cuba, which were capable of striking the American homeland within minutes of launching.

In Britain, the Campaign for Nuclear Disarmament (CND) was formed in February 1958. This became the most prominent nuclear disarmament group, campaigning on a unilateralist platform, which between 1960 and 1961 was also part of the Labour Party manifesto. In 1960 a group of activists, impatient with CND's legalistic electoral approach to nuclear disarmament, split from CND to form the Committee of 100. Led by Bertrand Russell and others, they took direct non-violent action in the form of mass civil disobedience as their form of protest.[43]

This increased awareness of nuclear issues prompted the formation, in the US, of an important medical peace organisation – the Physicians for Social Reponsibility.

PHYSICIANS FOR SOCIAL RESPONSIBILITY

In the US there was little opposition from the medical profession to their government's policy on nuclear weapons and civil defence. This was to change in 1960 when Dr Bernard Lown and a few colleagues heard Lord Noel-Baker (Nobel Peace Prize winner in 1959) speaking on the arms race and other nuclear issues at Cambridge, Massachusetts. In his speech he suggested a special role for physicians in peacemaking processes. Lown said of this lecture:

> Listening to him talk like some Hebraic Prophet, I felt profoundly shaken by my simplistic notion that the world would continue because it had done so up to now. He outlined the nuclear dilemma confronting humankind and clearly showed the crossroads we had reached. . . one fork the direction of unprecedented catastrophe.[44]

After this meeting Lown and a group of physicists and physicians began to meet regularly at his home, and 'struggled' to acquire some expertise in the field of nuclear war, nuclear weapons and civil defence. They formed the Physicians for Social Responsibility (PSR) in 1961, and in May 1962 as a result of the work of a committee representing the Special Study Section of the PSR[45] a collection of papers was published in the *New England Journal of Medicine*.[46] In the introduction to this seminal piece of work the question is asked: Why should physicians also be especially involved in the problem of nuclear war? The answers are clear:

> No single group is as deeply involved in and committed to the survival of mankind. No group is as accustomed to the labor of applying practical solutions to life-threatening difficulties. Physicians are aware, however, that intelligent therapy depends on accurate diagnosis and a realistic appraisal of the problem. The object of these articles is therefore the presentation to physicians of some of the facts of thermonuclear warfare.[47]

The group studied in some detail a scenario of a nuclear attack totalling 56 megatons targeted on Boston and the southern New England area of Massachusetts. These studies showed that previous efforts by the US Congress[48] underestimated the extent of death and destruction to be expected after a nuclear war, and they questioned the efficacy of civil defence preparations. PSR researchers and others had also linked Strontium 90 from radioactive fallout resulting from atmospheric nuclear testing, to that which was being found deposited in cows' milk, bones of children and infants' teeth.[49] The theme behind all the papers (other than their technical details) is that in the instance of nuclear war 'prevention is the only effective therapy'. The authors expressed the hope that physicians would 'carefully consider the implications of the articles for their role as physicians in a nuclear age and will be stimulated to play a greater part in the search for peaceful alternatives to thermonuclear war'. In 1963 a book of collected articles was published.[50]

The work of PSR helped create public pressure demanding a ban on atmospheric testing. In 1963 the Partial Test Ban Treaty was signed between the US, UK and USSR which halted atmospheric and underwater tests and prohibited testing in outer space by the signatory countries. PSR is committed to transforming the ways in which the medical community and the general public perceive nuclear weapons, and thereby contributing to the development of policies that will diminish the risk of mass destruction, while strengthening national and global security. PSR today believes that:

> Over the long term, nuclear war can only be prevented through

co-operative multilateral measures. The important differences between US and Soviet societies must be subordinated to our mutual self-interest in survival.[51]

DECLINE IN ANTI-NUCLEAR ACTIVITY BY THE PEACE MOVEMENT

After the signing in 1963 of the Partial Test Ban Treaty, the 'urgency' of nuclear weapons campaigning was removed. The Vietnam War and civil rights issues overshadowed 'nuclear tensions' in the US and elsewhere, and many medical activists started working in fields such as the anti-draft campaign and human rights issues. This slowdown was also reflected in Britain.

Paul Boyer identified five main reasons for the decline in nuclear awareness between 1963 and the end of the 1970s which affected all peace organisations.[52] These were:

1. Perception of diminished risk: partly due to various treaties such as SALT 1, NPT, PTBT, which conveyed the appearance of progress, even if in actuality they did fail to halt the arms race and to bring about a thaw in the cold war.
2. Loss of immediacy: memories of Hiroshima and Nagasaki dimmed. After a great emphasis on civil defence (CD) between 1948 and 1963[53] the government began to play down CD plans. The public was becoming 'familiar' with the bomb. The abstract terminology of the nuclear strategies and their array of nuclear acronyms (such as ALPS, BAMBI, MIRV, ASAT, etc.) and the names manufacturers gave to the missile systems (such as Bullpup, Poseidon, Davy Crockett, Hound Dog) 'evoked not their actual doomsday potential but reassuring associations with the heavens, classical mythology, American history and even popular slang', and furthered the loss of immediacy between these years.
3. The neutralising effect of the 'peaceful atom': domestic nuclear power was propagandised as a means of cheap, safe and limitless energy.
4. Nuclear apathy linked to the complexity and reassurance of nuclear strategy. In discussing this factor Boyer makes the important point that:

    ... deterrence theory as publicised in the later 1960's clearly reinforced the 'psychic numbing' process for many Americans. Once each side had achieved a credible second-strike capability (McNamara's 'Mutual Assured Destruction') the nuclear arms race would end in a tie. Nuclear warheads would remain, but they would simply rest in their silos and submarine bays forever, endlessly deterring.

5. The effects of the Vietnam War and the rise of the New Left. From the major escalation of February 1965 to the final evacuation of Saigon ten years later, the Vietnam War 'ruled the media and obsessed the national consciousness'. The bomb was a potential menace; Vietnam was an actuality. The New Left movement emerged from the campus-based radical organisations, particularly the Students for a Democratic Society. This generation had grown up with the bomb and they proposed a general indictment of capitalist society as a whole as the cause for the present threat of nuclear annihilation. Major social concerns overshadowed the menace of nuclear war.

MAPW IN THE 1960s AND 1970s

MAPW continued working mainly through organising a series of conferences. These were usually reported favourably in the press, and their proceedings occasionally published in an attempt to reach a wider audience.[54] Topics included: Psychological factors in war (1969); Medicine in North Vietnam (1967); Medicine in South Africa (1973); Education and war (1963); a biological approach to the problems of war (1964); and, Security has become a new problem (1966). This wide range of topics reflects MAPW's broad approach to studying peace, conflict and war.

In the Netherlands, during this time of reduced anti-nuclear concern, the Netherlands Association for Medical Polemology (NVMP) was founded towards the end of the 1960s. The main focus of NVMP campaigning was the Vietnam War and when this ended NVMP went into hibernation until 1980, when, along with other peace groups, it revived on the crest of a new wave of public opinion.[55]

As we shall now see, this period of relative inactivity around antinuclear issues was to end at the close of the 1970s with the re-emergence of nuclear concern as a major campaigning thrust for the peace movement.

RE-ACTIVATION OF THE PEACE MOVEMENT TO NUCLEAR ISSUES

In 1978, Dr Helen Caldicott,[56] a pediatrician working in Boston, rejuvenated Physicians for Social Responsibility (PSR) in the US. Before emigrating to America she had been a leading anti-nuclear activist in Australia, having led successful campaigns against French atmospheric testing in the South Pacific, and uranium mining in northwest Australia. In 1978 she published *Nuclear Madness*[57] which had some impact in the anti-nuclear movement. The newly active PSR at first concentrated on nuclear power, linking it with nuclear weapons and environmental damage. In 1979 PSR organised a major conference which, by coincidence, took place shortly after the accident at Three Mile Island nuclear power plant that almost resulted in a 'melt-down' of the reactor's core. Consequently, their meeting received good support from the press, public and medical profession.

Between 1979 and 1980 PSR's national focus shifted from nuclear power to nuclear weapons (for reasons behind the renewed interest in nuclear weapons, see below) and they held a second conference at Harvard on the theme of 'nuclear war and medicine'. One of the results of this was the publication of an open letter in the *New York Times* in 1980 which was signed by many well-known doctors appealing to Presidents Carter and Brezhnev to end the nuclear arms race. This was quite an extraordinary thing for a 'conservative' group such as the medical profession to do, and it could not be written off by the American administration as a protest by some pro-Soviet, left-wing organisation.

INTERNATIONAL PHYSICIANS FOR THE PREVENTION OF NUCLEAR WAR

During 1979, Bernard Lown (one of the founder members of PSR in the early 1960s and now an eminent cardiologist) approached Dr Evgeny Chazov,[58] a Soviet cardiologist and personal physician to Brezhnev. Lown and Chazov were friends as a result of professional meetings over the previous decade and Lown suggested that the time was perhaps appropriate for something to be done, by them, to help stop the arms race. In 1980 Lown went to Moscow, met with Chazov, and they agreed to organise an international conference to discuss the foreseeable medical consequences of nuclear war and the arms race. On his return to the US, Lown and a few colleagues incorporated International Physicians for the Prevention of Nuclear War (IPPNW) as a non-profit making and educational organisation. Day and Waitzkin[59] report that IPPNW emerged as a separate organisation from PSR partly because some PSR leaders, at that time, opposed close links with the Soviet medical profession. Members were uncomfortable with the role that some of their Soviet colleagues were playing in the abuse of human rights, by committing dissidents to psychiatric hospitals for 'rehabilitative' treatment.

Later in 1980 a group of US and USSR physicians (including Lown and Chazov) met in Geneva to formulate the policies of IPPNW.[60] These were:

1. That IPPNW would restrict its focus to nuclear war and the nuclear arms race.
2. That through IPPNW, physicians would work to prevent nuclear war as a consequence of their professional commitments to protect life and preserve health.
3. That IPPNW would involve physicians from around the world.
4. That the same information about nuclear war would be circulated widely to the public and leaders of all nations.
5. That although IPPNW might advocate certain steps to prevent nuclear war, it would maintain a neutral, non-partisan character.[61]

From its inception several factors indicated that IPPNW would be successful. It enjoyed the support of a respectable, upper middle class, 'conservative' group, and was not 'tainted' with any pro-Soviet bias by the US establishment. Importantly, there was initial high-level personal contact between Lown and Chazov, so that a large degree of mutual trust was already present. It has so far remained an anti-nuclear organisation with well-defined aims and objectives and has quite successfully managed to maintain a neutral stance with respect to superpower politics. There is, however, growing pressure from affiliates belonging to non-nuclear powers for increasing involvement by IPPNW in broader campaigning issues such as chemical and biological weapons and environmental concerns.

John Humphrey wrote of doctors' influence on the public:

> Even though doctors are often criticised, their standing as a whole

remains high in the public eye and they are regarded as solid and basically conservative citizens, not given to irresponsible criticism of government action ... when a substantial proportion of doctors are moved to make common cause over some issue their views are newsworthy, and indeed the media have given wider publicity to the activities of the physicians' organisations than to other groups of comparable size.[62]

Finally, IPPNW was incorporated at a time when anti-nuclear sentiment was peaking. In 1985 IPPNW was awarded the Nobel Peace Prize for:

> ... performing a considerable service to mankind by spreading authoritative information and by creating an awareness of the catastrophic consequences of nuclear war.[63]

This was a well-deserved international recognition of its contribution to world peace. Unfortunately, many Western governments criticised the award, mostly because of Chazov's alleged involvement in human rights abuses in the Soviet Union. The following adverse comment is typical: 'Headed by a Kremlin stooge and a naive American, the IPPNW is a bogus organisation doing more for Soviet propaganda than for peace.'[64] IPPNW responded by restating its founding principles and said that, just because it did not campaign as an 'organisation' for human rights, it did not condone abuses in this area *in any country*. Its success had been in maintaining a strict non-partisan view in working to eliminate the common enemy of all mankind – the nuclear weapon. By 1989 IPPNW had affiliates in 72 countries, a remarkable achievement.

MEDICAL CAMPAIGN AGAINST NUCLEAR WEAPONS (UK)

In the UK there was also growing awareness and opposition to nuclear weapons from the medical profession. In 1980 Dr Helen Caldicott spoke at meetings of doctors and others throughout Europe, encouraging the initiation of organisations with similar aims to PSR and IPPNW. Due to this activity the Medical Campaign Against Nuclear

Weapons (MCANW) was formed in Britain.[65] MCANW's stated aims were:

> ... to educate the profession and public about the foreseeable short-term medical consequences and uncertain long-term environmental and social effects that would result from the use of nuclear weapons in the expectation that this would lead to political pressure on govenment to abjure the threat of using nuclear weapons as an instrument of policy.[66]

Membership grew rapidly. There appear to have been several factors which reinvigorated medical peace activists (and recruited new members) and others in the years 1979–80. These included:

1. Development and purchase of new weapons systems (e.g. the British government decided to replace Polaris submarines with the new Trident types) and particularly the change from countercity to counterforce systems. These decisions were seen to aggravate and fuel the arms race. The new weapons were prompting a change in military strategy, and there was discussion in military circles and civilian policy institutes of developing methods of actually fighting and winning a nuclear war.[67]
2. Both horizontal and vertical proliferation seemed to be accelerating.
3. Agreement to deploy Cruise and Pershing II missiles (which were seen to be capable of first strikes) by 1983, coupled with the political and strategic implications entailed in those decisions.[68] Europeans realised very quickly that their homelands were to be the site for a future nuclear exchange by the superpowers:

    > ... we fought World War 1 in Europe, we fought World War 2 in Europe, and if you dummies let us, we'll fight World War 3 in Europe.[69]

4. Failure of the US Senate to ratify the SALT II Treaty and the issue of Carter's Presidential Directive 59, which defined the twin notions of 'limited nuclear war' and 'counterforce'.[70]
5. The British government's own public information leaflet on civil defence (CD), *Protect and Survive*,[71] received much criticism for its simplistic ideas and ineffectual advice. An editorial in *The Lancet*

voiced doubts about how truthfully the British public was being informed about the true extent of destruction after a nuclear war and referred to the CD exercise 'Operation Square Leg' which had been carried out earlier in the year.[72]

6. In Britain the existence of a DHSS circular, HDC(77),1[73] laying out the government's CD plans for the health services in time of nuclear war, came to light. Until then few doctors had heard of this, and fewer were involved.
7. Launching of the World Disarmament Campaign (WDC) as a result of the decisions of the United Nations Special Sessions on Disarmament in 1978.[74]
8. Election of perceived 'hawkish' governments both in the US and UK heightened nuclear tensions.

MCANW was not set up in opposition to MAPW, but as a single issue campaigning group. MAPW had traditionally not taken on such a public image, being committed to broader concerns of peace and justice and the study of war prevention. MCANW tapped into the strong sentiments of insecurity and doubt that had been stimulated by the factors mentioned above. MCANW and MAPW became the British affiliates of IPPNW.

How did the British medical 'establishment' respond to the newly active medical peace activists and their calls for it to take some stand on these concerns? In the next section we will look particularly at the response from the BMA.

BRITISH MEDICAL ASSOCIATION AND ITS RELATIONS WITH MAPW AND MCANW

As a response to the concern shown by some of its members, the British Medical Association (BMA), to which most doctors in the UK belong, instructed its Board of Science and Education, chaired by Sir John Stallworthy, to prepare a report on the medical effects of nuclear war. This was published in 1983 and thoroughly investigated the scenario after a nuclear attack on the UK, particularly considering the morbidity and mortality consequent to such an event.[75] Although they stated that 'each reader will make up his own mind on matters connected with the nuclear debate', their findings implicitly damned the current nuclear policy and the tasks set, by the government, for CD planners. The report stated that:

> ... the unreliability of basic assumptions has been a constantly recurring problem in all areas of our investigations. (p. 121)

and,

> The NHS could not deal with the casualties that might be expected following the detonation of a single one megaton weapon over the UK ... we believe that the provision of individual and medical or nursing attention for victims of a nuclear attack would become remote. At some point it would disappear completely and only the most primitive first aid services might be available from a fellow survivor. (p. 124)

The authors also thought that society and its values would not survive such a war. The BMA Report, which undoubtedly had great influence within the profession and peace movement, was, as could be expected, not popular with the government of the day who labelled it 'CND propaganda' and 'alarmist'. With the publication of the report the public had an impartial view of the dreadful aftermath of a nuclear war, clearly demonstrating the flaws and faulty assumptions (whether deliberate or not) upon which government planning was based.

THE BMA AND THE POLITICAL IMPLICATIONS OF THE 1983 REPORT

The report from the BMA's Board of Science and Education was debated at the 1983 BMA Annual Representative Meeting (ARM). In presenting it to the representatives, the BMA Council emphasised that '... approval of publication of the report must not be interpreted as the expression of any view of the politics of nuclear armament or disarmament'.[76]

Josephs records that the Agenda Committee for this meeting proposed a motion of its own recommending that: *the Association take no political stance*. According to BMA lawyers, 'political stance' meant anything relating to the British government's policy concerning the manufacture, testing and deployment of nuclear weapons. This motion was carried by the ARM which effectively meant that the BMA itself could not actively support IPPNW – its reports could only offer reliable *facts* for public information. The BMA would not take part in IPPNW's campaigning activities.[77]

Steve Watkins in his book *Medicine and Labour: The Politics of a Profession*[78] writes that the phrase 'no political stance' had such a deep emotional resonance for the delegates to the 1983 ARM when it was debating the question of nuclear war, because politics is seen as disuniting the medical profession:

> ... medical politics itself is depoliticised. It centres on conflicts between interest groups within the profession (such as juniors vs. consultants) and on the careers of individual medical politicians. It does not primarily involve conflicts in *ideas and values*.[79] (my emphasis)

Watkins goes on to say that this depoliticisation of medicine does not just serve internal purposes. It is also important for external consumption, in that doctors derive their status and power from their perceived independence.

The relationship between anti-nuclear activists (mostly MCANW and MAPW members), some of whom promote a more radical (even 'CND') line, and older, more conservative members within the BMA remains uneasy. David Josephs quotes a spokesman at the 1985 ARM:

> The BMA is not the organisation we joined. We are all now a pill-pushing, rent-a-womb, unilaterally disarming bunch of hippies![80]

Despite the BMA's 'no political stance', the 1984 and 1985 ARMs supported motions calling for 'a massive and progressive reduction in world arms spending, both nuclear and conventional' (1984) and a 'major change in the balance of government spending' (1985) in relation to diverting money from the armaments industries to health care and welfare at home and in developing countries.

In 1984 an international group of experts appointed by the World

Health Organisation (WHO) echoed the findings of the BMA in a report of their own.[81] They also stated:

> As doctors and scientists the members feel that they have both the right and duty to draw attention in the strongest possible terms to the catastrophic results that would follow any use of nuclear weapons.[82]

Both the BMA and WHO reports provided strong ammunition for anti-nuclear activists, particularly when campaigning against the current civil defence plans.

CIVIL DEFENCE PLANS: REACTION FROM THE MEDICAL PEACE MOVEMENT

Until the publication of the articles by Sidel *et al.*[83] the truth about the awesome consequences of nuclear war was not understood in the medical world, and thinking on these matters was, with hindsight, naive. With the 1980s and the renewed educational campaigning on the matter of CD by peace activists, the reality of the aftermath of nuclear war actually began to sink in. (Discovery of the effects of a possible 'nuclear winter' were to reinforce their efforts.) Ike wrote:

> The impotence of medicine thus demonstrated (in the Sidel article) has never been refuted on basic points since. It is still the *paradigma* in discussion on the role of medicine in nuclear war.[84]

Until then concern was for prevention of human suffering *after nuclear war, rather than working to prevent it*. The next few paragraphs will look at the case of CD in the United Kindgdom. For a summary of the US medical profession's attitude to CD see the work by Roth,[85] Leaning,[86] and Day and Waitzkin.[87]

The Role of Community Physicians

In Britain it was the community physicians who were given the responsibility to provide medical advice, to prepare an NHS plan and to learn and teach about nuclear war. A study group was set up in 1982 to review the implications of nuclear weapons for community medicine in terms of the immediate casualties, health service planning, CD, the longer term problems, and education in these areas.[88] The report produced contained the terms:

> ... the potential scale of damage to human life is so vast that there is a danger of an otherwise responsible profession simply looking the other way. Furthermore, there is a profound conflict between responsibilities to professional and personal ethics.

The Faculty of Community Medicine also called the issue 'the most important challenge to prevention in history'.

It is in the area of CD, which was renamed Civil Protection (CP) in 1986,[89] that some of the most effective lobbying and research work has been undertaken by the physicians' peace movement. Careful critiques have been produced of various government planning circulars and consultative documents on CD/CP measures in the NHS.[90] MAPW and MCANW published a booklet in 1982, *The Medical Consequences of Nuclear War*, which attempted to give a realistic account of a nuclear attack and its consequences.

Doctors fell into two camps: those who supported the government with active involvement in CD/CP planning in all its aspects,[91] and those who were more sceptical of government claims, particularly when it came to nuclear war planning.[92] The renewed debate on CD in the early 1980s was partly sparked off by a letter in *The Times* by Michael Howard, Professor of History at Oxford.[93] He wrote of the necessity of adequate CD measures to protect a 'substantial' number of the population in the event of a 'limited nuclear strike' by the Russians, particularly against the proposed Cruise missiles to be stationed in Britain. He felt that CD was an indispensable element of deterrence so that:

> ... the credibility of our entire defence posture should not be destroyed through the absence of evidence of our capacity to endure the disagreeable consequences likely to flow from it.

(One result of this letter was E. P. Thompson's *Protest and Survive*,[94] which was a forceful response to the assertions and speculations in Howard's letter and also to the pamphlet *Protect and Survive*[95] issued by the government.)

Both camps claimed the moral high ground. While accepting that nuclear war would be horrific, that prevention should be our top priority, and that total nuclear disarmament should be the ideal, Kersley, who was the chairman of the Conservative Medical Society and so supported the government's nuclear deterrent policy and 'peace through strength' stratagem, wrote: 'I believe that abrogation of medical responsibility (to CD), however difficult the situation, would be to break the Hippocratic Oath.'[96]

It was inexcusable, he thought, to refuse to do what one can to mitigate the resulting suffering of the victims. Conservative doctors called for an end to 'defeatist' attitudes and 'disarmament at any price' when it was simple to reduce casualties and curb disease by easy and inexpensive methods.[97]

Taking a different stand, Sepping[98] thought that CD should not be entirely discounted, and should continue to be seen as an ethical responsibility, but he disagreed with Kersley on the way planning for conventional war and natural disasters was lumped in with planning for nuclear war. What must be avoided is self-deception in the form of 'wishful thinking', which occurs in an atmosphere of maximum terror (as in the threat of mutual assured destruction), and where there is little opportunity for reality testing. Sepping postulated that, in small, densely populated Britain, the size of today's nuclear threat creates responses where delusional thinking can easily dominate. A belief in effective CD may induce a sense of false security which may in turn direct attention from the fundamental problem of East–West mistrust. CD in a thermonuclear situation becomes a *psychological necessity* in an atmosphere of nuclear terror.

Faculty of Community Medicine

In June 1988 the Faculty of Community Medicine provided a strongly worded statement on the issue of peace.[99] Based on the Alma Ata Declaration[100] and the WHO Report,[101] it identified peace as a vital underlying prerequisite of the Health for All goal and, in defining peace, stated:

> Peace is not just the absence of war. It is also a positive sense of well being for the people of all countries, implying the opportunity to freely determine their own destiny and fully exploit their

human potential... in Europe, at the present time, it is not war itself that presents health problems, but the fear of war.

The statement supported the concept of citizen diplomacy initiatives,[102] a massive reduction in arms spending, and international co-operation with peace initiatives.

DISAGREEMENT OVER CASUALTY CALCULATIONS

There had always been disagreement about casualty figures between the Home Office Scientific Research and Development Branch (SRDB) and professional peace movement groups such as MCANW and Scientists Against Nuclear Arms (SANA). SANA adapted figures from the US Office of Technology Assessment (OTA), which were more realistic and truthful in their estimation of post-nuclear attack damage. As a result government CD planners underestimated casualty numbers, the magnitude of the damage and the post-attack condition of society, and therefore underestimated the medical requirements which would be needed. Sepping felt that CD:

> ... is concerned with allaying fears about the aftermath of thermonuclear war by implying the return of Western-style medicine and also by ignoring the environmental sequelae of thermonuclear exchange.[103]

Recently (1989) the SRDB has revised its figures[104] so that they are nearer to those of SANA[105] and the OTA.[106] Holdstock noted:

> ... a widespread impression that SRDB estimates of the effects of a nuclear attack attempt to minimise casualty rates in order to make CD for a nuclear war, and hence current military strategies, seem credible.[107]

In the information booklet *Civil Protection*[108] and in the most recent (1988) DHSS planning circular HC(88)31, which was virtually the same as the document – HC(77)1 – it replaced, no mention was made of the possibility of a 'nuclear winter'[109] and associated environmental degradation.[110] Other criticisms made by groups such as MAPW and

MCANW, of HC(88)31, were that: it did not give any guidance on chemical weapons; it did not give any specific attack scenarios to work on; and ethical problems were not addressed. The ethical problems involved were, however, discussed by the BMA that year.

ETHICAL QUESTIONS FOR DOCTORS IN CONSIDERING NUCLEAR WAR

In 1988 the BMA attempted to address the ethical problem of priorities for treatment among survivors, in the forum of the BMA 'SNAC' Report.[111] Part 1 of the report updated the BMA report of 1983[112] and Part 2 considered how casualties might be selected for treatment. In disaster and mass casualty situations a method called 'triage' is used for allocation of medical resources to those in need. Casualties are sorted according to severity of illness (need) and priority for treatment (allocation).[113] In peacetime emergencies there is usually adequate backup, from on-site services and also outside agencies, to ensure eventual treatment for all casualties. In nuclear war this would not be the case. Not only will medical provisions be of a basic type, they will be extremely limited in availability. Doctors and other health workers will have to select those 'suitable for saving'. The difficult question of what criteria should be used has been a subject of much debate. The SNAC Report lays down the basic principles of treatment, attempting to list priorities (dependent on available resources), and advises that there must be no racial, political or religious bias. That this has to be spelt out, to doctors, is comment in itself. But it also says that food and health care priority would be given to children and previously 'healthy' young adults, particularly those with skills in agriculture and construction.

Controversially, the report advocates more training for lay people in the type of first aid that would be appropriate in the circumstances, and also training in immediate care for doctors – whilst admitting that for major injuries this would be no more than palliative. This aspect of the report was criticised by IPPNW on the grounds that:

1. It can be seen as sanctioning the physician's role in contingency planning for nuclear war and as endorsing government priorities for selecting whom to treat.

2. IPPNW has historically taken the position that there can be no adequate response to the consequences of a nuclear attack: where no remedy exists, prevention is the only cure.[114]

Haines et al., after reviewing the medical response to nuclear weapons, evaluated their potential risks and benefits and concluded:

> ... we believe that it is impossible to exclude the possibility of nuclear war, and that consequently support for either the continual build-up of weapons of mass destruction or for nuclear deterrence as credible policy for global security is incompatible with medical ethics.[115]

Nuclear deterrence, with the dreadful consequences should it fail, contravenes the overriding principle that doctors should be concerned with reasonable preservation of life, which carries the corollary that they should neither cause harm nor support policies which inflict harm on patients.

In discussing DHSS civil defence plans, Haines raises several ethical issues. Part of the planning envisaged the dispersion of health professionals. Should their priorities be to their families and local community or to the 'health district' in event of nuclear attack? It is suggested that doctors should not enter areas of high radioactive contamination to treat survivors, but Haines believes that 'such a principle appears to violate the responsibility of doctors to attend their patients even at personal risk, and should surely be left to conscience' (if their family was in such an area, would there by any choice?).

On the topic of triage the question asked is: should medical staff conserve supplies until the population has fallen enough to more 'manageable numbers', and then intervene medically? Should doctors consider large-scale euthanasia, knowing that many would die anyway after protracted suffering? In *The Doctor's View on War*[116] concern was voiced about the relationship between doctors and the policy of the state. Haines echoes this concern and points out that ethics appear never to have defined in detail 'the relationship between the conscience of the individual doctor and the political pressures of society in which he lives'. There are many countries in the world where doctors cooperate with the state by actively torturing prisoners; by helping to develop chemical and biolgical warfare techniques; or, as was the case, for example, in the USSR, by committing dissidents to mental institutions for political offences against the state.

Verdoorn in his book *Mars en Aesculapius*[117] concentrates on the structural disparity between civilian morals and military normatives. Military normatives are impervious to criticism based on civilian morals. Attempts to outlaw certain types of weapons are therefore foredoomed to failure. For the medical profession this means that any physician involved in military service must choose between the inalienable postulate of medical ethics (i.e. to save life) and conversion to an outlook characterised by Kimble Young as the exclusive basis of military morals – 'a complete and zealous faith in one's country and the war it is fighting'.

Some attempts have been made to formalise ethical and moral considerations in a manner which reflects the changed ethical, pragmatic, social and political realities since Hippocrates drew up his Oath.[118]

CONTRIBUTIONS FROM PSYCHIATRY AND PSYCHOLOGY TO THE NUCLEAR DEBATE AND PROMOTION OF PEACE

From 1945 psychiatrists and psychologists have continued their tradition of contributing to the debate on the causes of war and conflict and how to promote peaceful processes, both as individuals and as members of the peace movement. Soon after the first atomic explosion it was noted that 'atomic energy has become a psychological problem'.[119] The literature on the psychology of peace and war is vast, and I intend to illustrate only the main avenues explored by the profession in relation to the work of the medical peace movement. For a good critical analysis of psychologists' work from 1945 to 1984 on nuclear war related problems, in a historical context, the paper by Morawski and Goldstein is useful.[120] Much of the pioneering work in this field can be traced to Frank,[121] Lifton[122] and Mack.[123]

Robert Holt[124] states that citizens and leaders must first change many faulty underlying assumptions (of which he lists 20) that are inherent in our thinking on current political and social matters, nuclear weapons, national security and modern warfare, if psychologists are to meet Einstein's challenge that '... a new type of thinking is essential if mankind is to survive and move towards higher levels'.[125]

How can psychologists and psychiatrists help?

Adam d'Heurle looks at four areas in which psychologists can 'help to clear the way towards a realistic, sane and peaceful view of the world'.[126] These are:

1. Language.
2. The myth of superiority and the inevitability of aggression.
3. Shaking the trust in the rationality of the social machine.
4. The need for clear, logical thinking about war and the preparation for war.

Nils Lavik[127] gives two levels at which psychology and psychiatry may be relevant in the peace–war issue:

1. *Individual level*
   - A political leader or military commander may become psychotic, with his/her ability to behave rationally becoming seriously affected.
   - A political leader may have an abnormal personality, i.e. some degree of pathology, without reaching the psychotic level, which may influence his/her political behaviour.
   - Normal political leaders or military commanders may have nervous breakdowns during stress situations, which again might disturb their skills and decision-making.
2. *Collective level*
   - Normal individuals may show abnormal and highly irrational behaviour in group settings.
   - Groups or nations may behave irrationally and pathologically.
   - Inter-group and international conflicts may escalate to wars through 'malignant social processes'.[128]

DEFENCE MECHANISMS: WHY WE ACCEPT THE BOMB

On the collective level, psychological working groups at the IPPNW World Congresses[129] have examined the psychological defence mechanisms which attribute to people's acceptance of the nuclear deterrent with all its associated implications. In an excellent paper David Menkes,[130] in a review of research into psychological defence mechanisms involved in maintaining or adjusting to the nuclear arms race, identifies 26 mechanisms. Although these mechanisms can have short adaptive value for the individual in protecting himself from such disturbing emotions as terror or guilt, they were also thought to increase the likelihood that nuclear war would actually occur, because they impaired the realistic perspectives of those who possess nuclear weapons. This prevented the development and use of measures that could take control of the arms race. The peace movement has used the research done on the subject of psychological defence mechanisms to illustrate the mechanics and dangers of the nuclear arms race. They include:

Denial The problem is regarded as being too big to do anything about. People expect leaders and 'experts' to deal with it. The weapons' effects appear so monstrous that anything which could ignite a possible nuclear war is termed 'incredible', inconceivable', etc. Professor H. Richter[131] talks of denial to this threat as being due to *habituation* – the fact that we have lived with nuclear weapons since the Second World War without anything actually happening has led to a deadening of our awareness. He also describes the phenomenon of *displacement,* which is the transference of the main cause of worry to another 'object'.

Drawing upon old ways of thinking Security is sought, in the face of this new threat, by responding in the traditional way, by developing even better weapons and increasing stockpiles, and from notions of strength dominated by the concepts of 'winning' and 'losing'. These thought patterns have, of course, been outmoded by the realities of nuclear weapons.

Stereotyping The enemy is seen in a distorted and degraded way, as someone who is completely evil, for example, President Reagan's 'evil empire' when speaking of the USSR. Bronfenbrenner[132] described, after a visit to Russia in 1961, how the Russians' distorted view of America was a *mirror image* of the American people's distorted view of Russia. James Thompson[133] in discussing this listed the themes Bronfenbrenner gave as this image of the enemy:

1. They are the aggressors.
2. Their government exploits and deludes their people.
3. The mass of their people are not really sympathetic to the regime.
4. They cannot be trusted.
5. Their policy verges on madness.

Both Russians and Americans were bewildered as to how such nice people could have such awful governments. Thompson finds it useful to show that these perceptions can also be cast in terms of attributions:
1. They started it first; we responded.
2. They broke their word; we adjusted our position.
3. They are offensive; we are defensive.
4. They invade; we peacekeep.
5. They talk peace, but plan war; we mean peace, but reluctantly must also plan war.

It is clear that these perceptions and attributions are *self-fulfilling* and *self-sustaining*.

Dehumanisation   To justify our image and hostility to the 'enemy' we must deny them any human value or worthy motives. By talking in terms of megatonnage, peripheral damage (civilian deaths) and so on, not only is appreciation of an enemy diminished, but also our own humanity. Erikson[134] proposes the developmental aspects of a dominant psychological and potentially maladaptive process he calls 'pseudospeciation' in analysing the potential destructiveness of inter-group/international conflict in the nuclear age.

The above four factors, and others, contribute to what has been termed *psychic numbing* – the facts are often acknowledged, but their emotional accompaniment is not. This is protective in the short term, but in the long term it is maladaptive. People feel completely helpless in the face of an apparently unsolvable problem. The anxiety created is so great that it causes apathy and despair. The omnicidal nature of nuclear weapons has rendered nuclear war obsolete as a viable means of resolving conflict, and 'deep down' everybody knows this.

A CRITIQUE OF PSYCHOLOGICAL APPROACHES TO PEACE AND WAR CONSIDERATIONS

David Ingleby[135] looks at the two paradigms which have been used by psychologists in discussing war and peace issues: the clinical (or mental health) paradigm and the social–psychological paradigm. His main criticism of these two models is that they have tended to pay attention to the psychological factors in isolation from the political, social and

Part Four: 1946–90

economic ones. In practice, he says, psychologists have claimed authority to speak on three main issues: the causes of the arms race, and the end of war in general; the effects of these; and ways of intervening to tackle the problem.

Clinical Approach

The clinical approach favoured by psychiatrists and clinical psychologists assigns the most important role to factors endogenous to the individual (such as the psychological defence mechanisms already discussed). What gets overlooked in this analysis are the cultural and social–structural aspects; the political and historical determinants of war; the role of economic factors; technology; the military–industrial complex; and the control of the public mind by the government and media. He sums up his main objections to this approach as follows:

1. Nuclear war is not a danger because people *feel* threatened, but because they *are* threatened.
2. The problem is not that people *feel* powerless, but that, to a large extent, they *are*.

The 'therapies' such as 'empowerment' of individuals offered by this clinical approach do not relate to the real world. We just do not have the power to influence world affairs. (But events in Eastern Europe in the last few months of 1989 show that people *can* become empowered to change radically the society in which they live.)

Social–Psychological approach

For Ingleby the social–psychological approach[136] has been represented by two main components: attitude research and conflict theory. He acknowledges that both of these can make extremely valuable contributions, but, he says, both contain persistent inadequacies which stem from their tendency to reduce societal or international processes to interpersonal ones, or to relations between small groups, and he comments:

> I'm sure the military–industrial complex would be delighted to hear that war is inevitable until we all learn to live in perfect harmony!

He concludes his paper by addressing the question of how to have a practical effect in the peacemaking process; whom do we want to influence, and how do we imagine we are going to do it? He feels that it is naive to think that just by propagating scientific insights we can automatically set the human race on a more rational path. He says:

> We have to see ourselves as political agents, and consider our effectiveness in a conscious and deliberate way. In this way, psychology will indeed lose its political innocence: now it is time to demonstrate that this innocence never really existed, except in the wishful thinking of the profession's apologists.

Lifton also supported popular political action as a means to promote both peace and individual mental health, as a means for psychological empowerment, by confronting the questions of nuclear war as being *political* and *historical* in addition to psychological perspectives.

As well as the psychoanalytically orientated writings of Frank and others, some psychologists were working primarily in the area of international relations. Doob,[137] Kelman,[138] Burton[139] and others began to develop new paradigms in conflict resolution and mediation theories, methods and techniques which evolved partly from social and clinical psychological bases. It is these areas that some groups within the medical peace movement are trying to promote.

MEDIATION AND CONFLICT RESOLUTION: DEVELOPING A NEW ROLE FOR PHYSICIANS AND OTHER HEALTH WORKERS IN PEACEMAKING PROCESSES

Physicians and other health workers can, through their collective dedication to the relief of suffering, prevention of disease and general welfare of their patients, cross transnational and intercommunal boundaries more easily than most groups of professional workers. They also have, through their work, an international network of contacts who may be prepared to help by providing information and support in mediatory initiatives. IPPNW and its affiliates, whose membership has already demonstrated its commitment to world peace and co-operation, constitute a valuable pool of potential mediators.[140] There may be situations when a properly resourced and trained team can intervene (by invitation or by offering their services) in a conflict situation as *neutrals* to help facilitate the removal of psychological barriers and so help bring belligerents together for meaningful talks. To achieve this it is necessary to train would-be mediators in the appropriate skills and techniques which have been developed, and into which research is continuing at centres all over the world. These skills can be applied in interpersonal and intercommunal situations, as well as in the international arena. MAPW in England is currently (1990) looking at how health workers may play a more active role in this rapidly developing field of peacemaking (mediation and conflict resolution) and this area of research will be the subject of another study by the present author.

CONCLUSION

The preceding pages have illustrated many of the factors which have motivated medical men and women to concern themselves with the issues of peace, war and justice. It was not our objective to provide full details of the history of the peace movement and of doctors' participation in it (this would in any case take many volumes), but merely to give a flavour showing the main phases of activity and some of the insights gleaned from them.

The involvement of physicians and other health professionals can be seen to have covered two main themes within the context of the peace movement as a whole:

1. Theory and research
2. Application of (1) through political and 'grass roots' activism

Some practitioners, such as Virchow and Nicolai, combined both strands in their work, often to considerable professional and personal disadvantage. One of the important features in describing the work of these individuals and organisations is that they may act as 'role-models' for new generations of peacemakers and peacebuilders. As with the rest of the peace movement, their engagement with peace concerns came from a variety of traditions (some innovative of their time) such as religious beliefs, political affiliation, pacifist ideals, feminism and women's suffrage, education and internationalism.

Most had decided to take a more wholistic view of their medical work; caring for the individual patient on reductionist terms was not enough. They felt that a wider professional commitment to the improvement of the quality of human life was needed, and this also meant understanding and trying to prevent the destructive elements of conflict – so that war could be banished from the repertoire of conflict resolution methods. What is remarkable is the similarity of the fundamental arguments for peace which have continued over the years. Medical peace activists have always linked war with disease, and peace with health. War causes and aggravates diseases such as gonorrhea, smallpox, typhoid, cholera, malaria and so on. Battles give casualties with severe injuries and disabilities. In the general population there is an increase in malnutrition (with its associated medical problems) and psychological disorders. Nuclear war results in radiation diseases (such as leukaemia) and genetic damage to future generations. Doctors have highlighted these aspects of war when talking of the need for peace. Other studies have described how some leaders have been affected by medical conditions which could have influenced their decision-making capability; for example, Idi Amin, once leader of Uganda, was reputed to suffer from syphilis.[1]

This medical tradition of involvement in these areas of peacemaking continues today with the work of IPPNW and its affiliates. IPPNW can be seen as the culmination of the dreams of men and women like Joseph Rivière and Maria Montessori who worked for a truly international medical peace organisation. In assessing the work of IPPNW Professor John Humphrey, a long-time medical peace activist and distinguished physician, wrote:

> Perhaps the most striking feature of IPPNW has been the way in which leading Russian and US physicians initially, and leading doctors from other communist and non-communist countries later, were able to work together with no official status and under no official auspices but with a common purpose...

and,

> Its [IPPNW's] function is to alter attitudes and to help create an atmosphere conducive to change and to taking practical steps which it advocates ... it succeeded uniquely in creating East–West co-operation at a level of citizen diplomacy at a time when this was not easy.[2]

It is difficult to assess the impact of an individual group on the political machinations of the world, but the campaign waged over the years, especially during the last decade, by IPPNW and its affiliates has brought to the public's attention, in a unique way, some important aspects and implications of the arms race and insights into the causes and prevention of war. By 'medicalising' the language of peace to illustrate their arguments, health workers have ensured a central role for themselves in the nuclear disarmament debate in particular.[3]

If nation states retain the *right* to wage war in settling disputes, then the hope of any sort of positive world peace will remain just a dream. So it is vital to look at alternative ways for nation states to resolve their conflicts, using what some authorities see as the new paradigms emerging in the field of conflict resolution. This also entails a major change in thinking, and of heart, within the anarchic system of international relations. These strategies must be based on solid academic models, be realistic, and offer acceptable political applications. Evidence must be shown that the old ways of carrying on power-based relations (win/lose) can be successfully replaced with the new paradigms of conflict resolution based on a win/win approach, resulting in long-term resolution of deep-rooted conflicts. Changes which have occurred in Eastern Europe, due mostly to the efforts of President Gorbachev and the processes of *glasnost* and *perestroika*, offer an opportunity for new administrations to look closely at how they may be able to act more effectively on the world stage – in a manner which will promote peaceful solutions to international disputes.

The medical peace movement recognises that it has a part to play in the developing field of conflict resolution. Health workers with their training, commitment to the well being of their patients, and situation are often well placed to facilitate initiatives. These can be on several levels of interaction.

Interpersonal: making contacts and breaking down barriers through exchange visits. Learning about human relationships (which are at the root of all conflict) and perfecting interpersonal skills, to help, for example, in effective communication.

Intercommunal: we live in a multi-racial community with all the tension that involves. Community Mediation Services help resolve disputes using non-violent conflict resolution techniques. Emphasis is laid on disputants taking on the responsibility to sort out their conflict with the objective of reaching a win/win agreement.

International: as has already been mentioned, doctors and others may be able to help in the resolution of major conflicts, through channels of non-official, third-party mediatory approaches – also known as 'track

Conclusion

two' or 'citizen' diplomacy. For example, they may be able to overcome difficulties of entry into the conflict and of obtaining access to the parties concerned (paticularly to insurgents) by demonstrating that their interest is purely humanitarian – to help stop further suffering by all parties and to provide treatment equitably to all parties.

In the field: Health workers are often at the point of conflict, whether in major wars or insurgency situations, and may be able to use mediatory *influences* to calm the situation or facilitate communications between belligerents. Skill and delicacy is required if mediation is attempted, so as not to jeopardise their primary task of medical care to the victims. It has been suggested that members of health teams working in the field for aid and development agencies may be in a position to influence the conflict process, but it must be remembered that acts of political insensitivity by well-intentioned, but poorly prepared and informed persons may result in worsening the situation.

To field workers it is often evident that a conflict is due to a major power imbalance between the belligerents. Many peace researchers and activists, like Galtung and Curle, feel that this element of the situation must be addressed with the same vigour as attempting to resolve or mediate the conflict – one way of doing this is finding means to empower the weaker party, without unacceptable cost to the more powerful party. However, it should be accepted that in some cases an imbalance is so marked that, in the perception of the oppressed party, resolution by peaceful methods is not realistic, and the methods and techniques involved in conflict resolution and mediation are just not appropriate.

So, how can non-government organisations (NGOs) and citizens become effectively involved in peaceful conflict resolving and mediatory processes, previously regarded as the sole domain of the professional politician and diplomat? Adam Curle and others have developed the conception of an international mediation network, into which NGOs such as IPPNW could fit. The network is seen to be composed of three main groups:

1. *Principal* network members, e.g. Secretaries-General of UN, OAS, Commonwealth and other large international organisations.
2. *The switchboard,* an intermediary group which scans and monitors

conflicts, serves as a referral and mediation service, confidential sounding board, etc.
3. *A group* composed of institutions, universities and NGOs (such as IPPNW and its affiliates and other professional groups) which would add scholarly research and practitioner or process experts as resources to the principal members.

This 'switchboard model' network would fill a void that currently exists in the resolution of conflicts by supplementing efforts of international organisations and other institutions by feeding in all the expertise available (but not so visible as the more 'eminent' persons and groups) from the *grass roots* level. An attempt has been made in this direction by The Conflict Resolution Programme, Carter Center of Emory University, Atlanta. Here an International Negotiation Network (INN) has been set up whose objectives are to monitor existing and emerging conflicts; spotlight conflicts that require third-party assistance; convene confidential consultations for disputants and mediators; mediate civil conflict; match disputants' needs with potential third parties, funding sources and experts, etc.

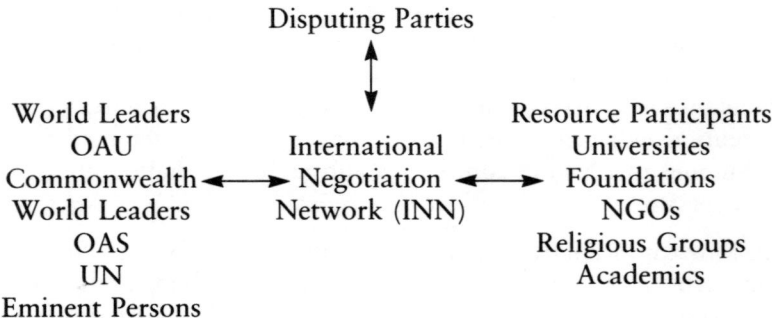

A paradigm shift is required in the way conflict is viewed (at all levels) from win–lose objectives to a greater global competence in operating techniques of win–win models. With a need for increasing international co-operation in environmental issues, which transcend national boundaries, and rapid political change the world over, the urgency of developing alternative strategies in non-violent, long-lasting resolution of conflict is becoming more apparent. These methods should involve as many people, from all levels of their own societies, as possible.

One suggestion proposed to help achieve the last-mentioned ambition is that of a UN Second Assembly. This idea of a subsidiary organ of the General Assembly, under Article 22 of the UN Charter, originated in MAPW's written statement to the UN Special Session on Disarmament in 1982[4] and is being promoted by the International Network for a UN Second Assembly (INFUSA). This Second Assembly would be concerned objectively with fundamental global problems: principles for world disarming; methods of making safer the inherited systems of international relations and security; problems of development, environment and so on. The Assembly would be composed of non-governmental delegates who would represent the peoples as *global inhabitants* and would thus complement our existing governmental representation in the UN General Assembly as *national citizens*.[5] The members would be ordinary people from all walks of life and it was proposed that the number of delegates from each country should be proportional to the square roots of national populations. This principle for representation and of voting power was proposed by Lionel Penrose (Chairman of MAPW, 1962–72, q.v.) in 1964.

In the past many theories and academic research findings, emanating from peace research institutions and anti-war groups, have not proved to be applicable to real-life situations – the international and diplomatic community and decision-makers around the world do not want to relinquish their hold on traditional means of dealing with conflict and potential conflict. It is vital that the new thinking in this area, and the role of citizens and NGOs in the developing field of 'track two diplomacy', address the issues in a hard-headed, feet-on-the-ground manner. The role of these latter groups should be seen to complement, not directly challenge, existing international relations channels, whilst the advantages of the alternative methods are given time to demonstrate their long-lasting benefits to conflict resolution.

Whilst the sweeping political changes which have occurred in Europe offer the opportunity for more peaceful dispute resolution mechanisms to be put in place (e.g. through the CSCE negotiations), new questions concerning the security roles of the US and the USSR have been posed. Also, the reassertion of national and ethnic identities is creating new sources of actual and potential conflict both within the

USSR itself and within the now independent nation states of Eastern Europe. Increasingly, the processes for change in these situations are becoming violent in nature.

Despite the signing of treaties such as the Intermediate Nuclear Force Treaty (INF) there remains a nuclear equivalent of three tons of dynamite for every human being on the planet. Nuclear modernisation continues unabated and there is a nuclear test every 8.7 days. Powerful media images have shown the concrete wall of Berlin slowly being chipped away, but the old walls of fear, mistrust and hate still remain in the hearts and minds of many of the world's decision-makers. World spending on armaments increases. In the 1989 edition of *World Military and Social Expenditures*[6] comparisons are made between world health needs and military spending. They include such alarming statistics as:

- Every minute 15 children die for lack of essential food and inexpensive vaccines, and every minute the world's military machine spends another $1.9 million in public funds.
- There is one physician for every 235 people in the USSR and in Burkina-Faso there is one for 53,933 people.
- 250,000 children go blind in the 'developing' world for lack of a 10 cent vitamin capsule.

What is evidently needed to correct the disgraceful disparity between the state of health of the affluent and that of the poorer members of the world community is a reorganisation of economic and moral priorities. Governments must change from being international arms traders to international health and peace traders. The responsibility also rests with countries receiving 'aid' – many of whom spend vast amounts in supporting armies and internal police forces for social control. Priority should be given to achieving the aims of the 1978 Alma Ata Declaration: Health for All by the Year 2000. This requires political change.

The need for international, transnational NGOs such as IPPNW is as acute as ever. There is still great danger from the use of nuclear weapons, and also increasing concern because of the horizontal proliferation of these weapons. Some countries are quite prepared to use chemical and biological weapons when this serves their purpose. Other tensions exist throughout the world, such as that between India and Pakistan over the Kashmir region – and both countries have nuclear

Conclusion

capabilities. Many members of the medical peace movement are worried about the complacency now pervading the world because of the perceived reduction of nuclear threat due to increasing co-operation and détente between the US and USSR. IPPNW, along with other campaigning groups, continues to lobby for a Comprehensive Test Ban Treaty (CTBT) as the major element needed to put an end to the nuclear arms race, and to bolster the increasingly fragile Non-Proliferation Treaty (NPT).

There is much debate within IPPNW and its affiliates as to what objectives and aims are relevant to the new security needs emerging in the world. If IPPNW is not to wither as an effective and vibrant organisation, the basis of dialogue among IPPNW and the peace movement, the medical profession, the general public, and decision-makers must be adapted to accord with prevalent concerns and the changing security requirements of the world's nations. This can be done whilst retaining its founding principle of opposition to nuclear weapons. With reference to this principle, Bernard Lown, co-president of IPPNW, has been reported as saying

> that since man's invention could not be disinvented, the world required permanent guardians who would sound the warning if the nuclear threat surfaced ... the health professions were duty bound to be such guardians.[7]

To illustrate how IPPNW is reacting can be seen by looking at their active programmes for 1990.[8] The three main thrusts of IPPNW activity are:

1. An International Test Ban Campaign – *Cease-Fire Now!* IPPNW's 'medical prescription' calls for an immediate end to all nuclear explosions and the negotiation of a comprehensive test ban treaty,
2. A Commission on the Health Costs of Nuclear Weapons Production. This commission was formed to investigate the environmental and human health effects of the nuclear weapons production cycle. Work undertaken includes studies on the health of people who have lived near nuclear bomb testing facilities and environmental damage in these areas.
3. The revolution in communication and space technology has made possible projects such as SatelLife. SatelLife when operational:

- will link isolated health workers to critical sources of information and consultation
- provide communication systems for relief efforts during natural disasters
- promote successful public health programmes by networking institutions and agencies
- interconnect medical libraries and research institutions
- gather data for surveillance and control of epidemic and endemic diseases
- offer computer-based learning programmes for field workers
- facilitate telebridging so that remote health sites can participate in medical symposia, meetings and conferences.

Other IPPNW activities have included the development of a model medical curriculum called 'Medicine and Nuclear War' which affiliates have been trying to get accepted for medical undergraduate teaching, and an International Physicians' Exchange network which helps to dispel the fears and stereotypes which have resulted from a lack of contact. In July 1990 IPPNW endorsed a boycott of General Electric (GE), which is the US's second largest nuclear weapons manufacturer.[9] GE also markets medical equipment (like CAT scanners) and, it was reasoned, if large orders of $500,000 or more could be blocked, 'even a corporate giant might sit up and take notice'. Zheutlin writes:

> In encouraging its 250,000 members to support the boycot, IPPNW cited GE's inconsistency in making both life-saving equipment and weapons of mass destruction . . . IPPNW believes that GE bears some responsibility for the adverse health and environmental consequences of its nuclear weapons operations.[10]

IPPNW hoped to persuade GE, and all nuclear weapons manufacturers, to re-examine their role in the military–industrial complex.

IPPNW is a successful transnational and international NGO, whose history and influences have been traced earlier in this book. Castillo[11] uses Robert Keohane's criteria to support the view that IPPNW is a catalytic international institution which provides leadership 'when individual incentives to co-operate are weak but the collective interest is strong'. IPPNW has provided, says Castillo,

1. Information to governments;

Conclusion

2. A secretariat which provides leadership by devising plans of action and lobbying governments for change;
3. A standard by which a government's performance and contribution to the common good and global health can be measured.

Although IPPNW is undoubtedly the focus for the medical peace movement, two other groups, in the UK, deserve mention at this point for the humanitarian and campaigning work they undertake, namely, the Medical Group of Amnesty International (which was formed to campaign on behalf of medical professionals who are harassed or wrongfully imprisoned, and to protest at the withholding of medical treatment for prisoners) and the Medical Foundation for the Care of Victims of Torture[12] which specialises in the treatment and support of torture victims from all over the world. The Medical Group of AI highlights two aspects of health carers and human rights.[13] First, health care professionals are frequently in the front line in the many countries where human rights are under attack. AI mentions Chinese hospital staff being shot in reprisals for showing television crews the dead and wounded after the Tiananmen Square massacre; death threats to leaders of the Chilean Nursing Association after they denounced dangerously poor health services; and more than 90 Syrian doctors detained since protests in 1980 for greater human rights.[14] Second, while many health workers put themselves in great danger simply by upholding professional standards of care, in some places professional ethics are being breached by the involvement of health personnel in the workings of repression. AI recounts instances where nurses have assisted in the amputation of the hands of thieves under Pakistan law; USSR dissidents have been detained in psychiatric hospitals; and neuroleptic drugs to induce pain have been used in torture in Uruguay.

Whatever priorities those involved in the medical peace movement decide are the most pressing to keep its members mobilised and also to maintain its unique identity, speaking of IPPNW and the future role for physicians Bernard Lown has said:

> The powerful voice of ordinary people throughout Europe has proved that a long overdue new agenda of humane priorities is possible. We speak as physicians with a spirit of hope and optimism. Only working together to end nuclearism and militarism can we at last begin to heal an ailing planet.[15]

NOTES

INTRODUCTION

1. James O'Connell, 'Towards an Understanding of Concepts in the Study of Peace' in J. O'Connell and A. Curle *Peace With Work To Do: The Academic Study of Peace* (Leamington Spa: Berg, 1985), p.50.

PART ONE

1. Adam Curle, 'Making Peace', *New Internationalist*, March 1983, p.27.
2. James O'Connell, 'Towards an Understanding of Concepts in the Study of Peace' in J. O'Connell and A.Curle, *Peace with Work to Do: The Academic Study of Peace* (Leamington Spa: Berg, 1985), p.30.
3. James O'Connell, *Making the Future: Thinking and Acting about Peace in Contemporary Britain* (UK: Trentham Books, 1989), p.24.
4. Charles Chatfield, 'Concepts of Peace in History', *Peace and Change*, Vol.XI, No.2, 1986, pp.11–21.
5. G.K. Wilson, *A Global Peace Study Guide* (London: Housmans, 1982), p.31; and also see N. Desai, *Handbook for Satyagrahis* (New Delhi: Gandhi Peace Foundation, 1980).
6. F. Beer, 'Just War', in L. Pauling (hon. ed.), *World Encyclopedia of Peace: Vol. 1* (London: Pergamon Press, 1986), pp.508–11.
7. Michael Banks, 'Conceptions of Peace', in Sandole and Sandole-Staroste (eds), *Conflict Management and Problem Solving. Interpersonal to International Applications* (New York University Press, 1987), pp.259–74.
8. A.C.F. Beales, *The History of Peace* (London: G. Bell & Sons, 1931), p.45.
9. Michael Howard, *War and the Liberal Conscience* (Oxford University Press, 1981), p.36.
10. James O'Connell (1989), op. cit., p.6.
11. Bob Overy, *How Effective Are Peace Movements?* (Montreal: Harvest House, 1982), p.2.
12. Taken from Nigel Young, 'Tradition and innovation in the British Peace Movement: towards an analytical framework', in R. Taylor and N. Young (eds), *Campaigns for Peace: British Peace Movements in the twentieth century* (Manchester University Press, 1987), pp.8–9.
13. See C. Horrie and P. Higgins, *Sanity*, November 1982, p.25. P. Allen, *Sanity*, June 1984, p.4. *Guardian*, 4 April 1983, article by David Pallister. *Guardian*, 8 October 1983, article by Susan Thomas.
14. P.P. Everts, *The Peace Movement and Public Opinion: Prospects for the Nineties*,

paper given at 30th International Studies Association Convention, London, 28 March–1 April, 1989.
15. From Nigel Young, op. cit., p. 12.
16. C. Mitchell, *The Structure of International Conflict* (London: Macmillan, 1981), in the introduction.
17. A. Mack, *Peace Research in the 1980's* (Canberra: Australian National University, 1985).
18. H. Newcombe and A. Newcombe, *Peace Research around the World* (Ontario: Canadian Peace Research Institute, 1972).
19. James O'Connell (1989), op. cit., p. 49.
20. David Dunn, 'Peace Studies', in L. Pauling (hon. ed.), *World Encyclopedia of Peace: Vol. 1* (London: Pergamon Press, 1986), pp. 247–51.
21. See n. 17.
22. Ibid.
23. See G. K. Wilson in n. 5.
24. Nigel Young, *Studying Peace: Problems and Possibilities* (London: Housmans, 1981).
25. J. Dedring, *Recent Advances in Peace and Conflict Research: A Critical Survey* (London: Sage Publications, 1976).
26. R. O. Moon, *The Relation of Medicine to Philosophy* (London: Longmans, Green and Co., 1909).
27. H. Joules (ed.), *The Doctor's View on War* (Woking: Unwin Bros, 1938). Chapter 7: Doctors on the Battlefield.
28. Quoted in Y. Sandoz, 'The Red Cross and Peace: Realities and Limits', *Journal of Peace Research*, Vol. 24, No. 3, 1987, p. 287.
29. A. Rosas, 'The Factors of Humanitarian Law', *Journal of Peace Research*, Vol. 24, No. 3, 1987, pp. 219–36.
30. J. Meurant, 'Inter Arma Caritas: Evolution and Nature of International Humanitarian Law', *Journal of Peace Research*, Vol. 24, No. 3, 1987, pp. 237–49.
31. A. Baccino-Astrada, *Manual on the Rights and Duties of Medical Personnel in Armed Conflicts* (Geneva: ICRC, 1982).
32. *The Geneva Conventions of August 12 1949*, (Geneva: ICRC, 1982). *Protocols additional to the Geneva Conventions of 12 August 1949* (Geneva: ICRC, 1977).
33. See n. 28.
34. ICRC. *To Promote Peace: Resolutions on Peace adopted by the International Movement of the Red Cross since 1921* (Geneva: ICRC, July 1986).
35. David Forsythe, 'Humanitarian Mediation by the International Committee of the Red Cross', in S. Touval and W. Zartman (eds), *International Mediation in Theory and Practice* (Boulder, Colorado: Westview Press, 1985), pp. 233–49.
36. A. R. Jonsen and A. J. Jameton, 'Social and political responsibilities of physicians', *Journals of Medicine and Philosophy*, Vol. 2, 1977, p. 380.
37. P. Lowinger, 'The Doctor as Political Activist', *American Journal of Psychotherapy*, Vol. 22, Oct. 1968, p. 623.
38. Notes from Ethical Subcommittee of Medical Association for the Prevention of War, 29 January 1987.
39. J. Geiger, 'Hidden Professional Roles: The Physician as Reactionary, Reformer, Revolutionary', *Social Policy*, Vol. 1, March/April 1974, p. 28.
40. C. Cassel and A. J. Jameton, 'Medical responsibility and thermonuclear war', *Annals of Internal Medicine*, Vol. 97, 1982, pp. 426–32.
41. M. McCally and C. Cassell, 'Medical Responsibility and Global Environmental

Change', *Annals of Internal Medicine*, Vol. 113, No. 6, 1990, pp. 467–73.
42. Ibid., pp. 467–8.
43. B. Lown, 'Physicians Confront the Nuclear Peril', *Circulation*, Vol. 72, No. 6, December 1985, p. 1141.
44. A. Relman, 'Physicians, Nuclear War and Politics', *New England Journal of Medicine*, Vol. 307, No. 12, 16 Sept. 1982.
45. Ibid., p. 745.
46. A. R. Jonsen and A. J. Jameton, op. cit., p. 377.
47. C. Cassel *et al.*, 'The Physician's Oath and the Prevention of Nuclear War', *Medicine and War*, Vol. 2, No. 1, 1986, pp. 51–6.
48. British Medical Association, *The Handbook of Medical Ethics* (London: BMA, 1981).
49. The Medical Group of Amnesty International has a particular interest in documenting such cases.
50. R. O. Moon, op cit., p. xi.

PART TWO

1. D. Allen, *The Fight for Peace, Vol. 1* (New York: Garland Publishing, 1971), pp. 245–7.
2. P. Lambert, 'Benjamin Rush: Physician in Politics', *Journal of Oklahoma State Medical Association*, Vol. 65, June 1972, pp. 218–24.
3. Franklin had been sent to England by the American colonists to protest against the Stamp Act of 1765.
4. *Common Sense* discussed the reasons for going to war with England. Paine, who had been forced to leave England in 1774 for 'agitation', arrived in Philadelphia with a note of introduction from Franklin in London. He later took part in the French Revolution of 1789 and wrote *The Rights of Man* (1791) and *The Age of Reason* (1794).
5. P. Lambert, op. cit., p. 220.
6. Ibid.
7. D. Malone (ed.), *Dictionary of American Biography. Vol. 7* (New York: Charles Scribner & Sons, 1935), pp. 227–31.
8. P. Lambert, op. cit., p. 222. Lambert quotes from a pamphlet published by Cobbett: *The Rush-Light*, New York, 28 February 1800, p. 49.
9. P. Lambert, op. cit., p. 223.
10. D. Malone, op. cit., p. 230.
11. D. Malone (ed.), *Dictionary of American Biography, Vol. 6* (New York: Charles Scribner & Sons, 1933), pp. 359–60.
12. H. Josephson (ed.), *Biographical Dictionary of Modern Peace Leaders* (London: Greenwood Press, 1984), p. 573. Article on George Logan.
13. J. Garraty and J. Sternstein (eds), *Encyclopedia of American Biography* (New York: Harper & Row, 1974), p. 682.
14. H. Josephson (ed.), op. cit., p. 573.
15. J. Garraty and J. Sternstein (eds), op. cit., p. 683. For a more recent account of examples of citizen diplomacy see G. Warner and M. Shuman, *Citizen Diplomats* (New York: Continuum Press, 1987).
16. J. McDonald, *Further Exploration of Track Two Diplomacy*. Paper given at

Notes

International Studies Association Conference, London, March 1989.
17. A.C.F. Beales, *The History of Peace* (London: G. Bell & Sons, 1931), p.45.
18. M. Howard, *War and the Liberal Conscience* (Oxford University Press, 1981), p.36.
19. A.C.F. Beales, op. cit., p.47.
20. Ibid. p.8..
21. Ibid. p.41.
22. M. Howard, op. cit., p.41.
23. A.C.F. Beales, op. cit., p.67.
24. Ibid. pp.94–116.
25. Ibid. p.105.
26. H. Josephson (ed.), op.cit. pp.994–5.
27. L. Eisenberg, 'Virchow: Physician as Politician', *Medicine and War*, Vol. 2, No.4, 1986, pp.243–50.
28. This was at the time when Henry Richard, the British MP and pacifist, was touring the Continent helping to inspire motions on disarmament in eight European parliaments. See A.C.F. Beales, op. cit., p.124. Richard met Virchow in Berlin.
29. L. Eisenberg, op. cit., p.245.
30. Quoted in L. Eisenberg, op. cit., p.245.
31. D. Pridan, 'Rudolph Virchow and Social Medicine in Historical Perspective', *Medical History*, Vol. 8, No. 1, 1964, pp.274–8.
32. L. Eisenberg, op. cit., p.244. This paper was originally read at the 6th International Physicians for the Prevention of War (IPPNW) Congress in Koln, FRG, 1986.
33. H. Josephson (ed.), op. cit., p.282.
34. A. Fischoff, 'On The Reduction of Continental Armies', in S. Cooper (ed.), *Arms Limitations* (New York; Garland Library of War and Peace, 1972), p.14. Article translated by H.W. Freeland.
35. Fischoff had in mind an organisation such as the Interparliamentary Union which was eventually formed in 1889.
36. A. Fischoff, op. cit., p.19.
37. S.E. Cooper, 'Women's Participation in European Peace Movements, The Struggle to Prevent WW1', in R. Pierson (ed.), *Women and Peace: Theoretical, Historical and Practical Perspectives* (London: Croom Helm, 1987), pp.51–75.
38. H. Josephson (ed.), op. cit., pp.527–8; M.A. Boxer, 'Socialism faces Feminism: The Failure of Synthesis in France, 1879–1914', in M. Boxer and J. Quataert, *Socialist Women* (New York, 1978), pp.75–111.
39. H. Josephson (ed.), op. cit., pp.966–7.
40. Ibid.
41. S.E. Cooper, op. cit., p.22.
42. C. LaVigna, 'The Marxist Ambivalence Toward Women: Between Socialism and Feminism in the Italian Socialist Party', in M. Boxer and J. Quataert, op.cit. pp.151–2.
43. C. LaVigna, op. cit., p.152.
44. Ibid. p.161.
45. H. Josephson (ed.), op. cit., p.527.
46. M. Boxer and J. Quataert, op.cit. p.103.
47. H. Josephson, op. cit., p.739.
48. M. Boxer and J. Quataert, op. cit., p.103.
49. H. Josephson (ed.), op. cit., p.740.

50. C. Chatfield, 'Concepts of Peace in History', *Peace and Change*, Vol. XI, No. 2, pp. 11–21, quoted at p. 16.
51. M. Boxer and J. Quataert, op.cit. p. 98.
52. Leo Tolstoy (1829–1910) believed in absolute non-violence as exemplified in Christ's Sermon on the Mount. When Jesus said 'Resist not him that is evil', Tolstoy interpreted this literally. He thought that every state was a slave state organised for the sole purpose of exploiting a subject population.
53. P. Brock, *Pacifism in Europe to 1914* (Princeton University Press, 1972), p. 468.
54. H. Josephson (ed.), op. cit., pp. 888–9.
55. A. J. Rivière, *Un Demi-Siècle de Physicotherapie. Organisation Mondiale de la Paix. Tome III* (Paris: Imprimerie et Libraire Centrales des Chemins de Fer, 1934), p. 209.
56. *The Lancet* of 8 April 1905, p. 945, gave the number of doctors who attended as 'over 200'. There were also many letters of support, including one from Professor Charles Richet who won the Nobel Prize for Physiology in 1913, and was a leading European pacifist of the time. See below.
57. A. J. Rivière, op. cit., pp. 214–16.
58. Ibid., p. 412.
59. The *Daily Telegraph*, 7 March 1906, listed such eminent British doctors as Sir Robert Cooper, Sir Francis McCabe, Sir William Thompson and Sir James Crighton-Browne as members. Collins was an MP (1906–10 and 1917–18), a member of the National Peace Council, and presided over the 5th British National Congress in Cardiff (1909).
60. A. Fried, *Handbuch der Friedensbewegung. Zweiter Teil. Verlag der 'Friedens-Warte'* (Berlin and Leipzig, 1913), p. 294. Fried incorrectly gives the year that IMAW was formed as 1904 and, from other evidence, his figure of 6,000 for the membership seems rather inflated.
61. From a speech given at Caxton Hall, London, 27 July 1908, and reported in *Official Report of the Seventeenth Universal Congress of Peace, 1908* (London: National Council of Peace Societies, 1909), pp. 94–5 and pp. 202–3.
62. A. J. Rivière, op. cit., p. 217.
63. A. J. Rivière, *Esquisse Clinique de Physicotherapie. (Traitement rationnel des Maladies Chronique). Tome II* (Paris: Editions Medicales, Norbert Malone, 1932).
64. Founded in 1980. See below.
65. H. Josephson (ed.), op. cit., p. 808.
66. Ibid.
67. Charles Richet, *L'Homme Stupide* (Paris: 1919). This was translated by Norah Forsythe and Lloyd Harvey as *Idiot Man or the Follies of Mankind* (London: T. Werner Laurie, 1925). It is from this edition that quotations from the book are taken.
68. Charles Richet, op. cit., p. 81.
69. Ibid., p. 140.
70. This was published as *International Language* (Warsaw: 1887). Zamenhof used the pseudonym Esperanto (one who hopes) to protect his medical career.
71. From *Die Friedens-Warte*, Berlin–Vienna, Vol. 14, Oct. 1912, pp. 391–2. This was the most important peace periodical of the German-speaking world at the time.
72. A. Fried, op. cit., p. 380 (Monnier); p. 384 (Nilsson); p. 390 (Polak).
73. Dr J. Polak, *A Short Contribution to the History of Pacifism in Poland*, published

by the Organising Committee of the XXVI Universal Peace Congress, Warsaw. No date, but after 1926.
74. A.C.F. Beales, op. cit., p.278.
75. Ibid.
76. N. Young, 'War Resistance and the British Peace Movement Since 1914', in R. Taylor and N. Young (eds), *Campaigns for Peace* (Manchester University Press, 1987), pp.23–48.
77. Ibid., p.33.
78. H. Josephson (ed.), op. cit., p.416.
79. V. Brittain, *The Rebel Passion: A Short History of Some Pioneer Peacemakers* (London: George Allen and Unwin, 1964), p.54.
80. Ibid., p.35.
81. H. Josephson (ed.), op. cit., p.416.
82. J. Vellacott, 'Women, Peace and Internationalism', in C. Chatfield and P. van den Dungen (eds), *Peace Movements and Political Cultures* (Knoxville: University of Tennessee Press, 1988), p.116.
83. S. Cooper, 'Women's Participation in European Peace Movements. The Struggle to Prevent World War I', in R. Pierson (ed.), *Women and Peace* (London: Croom Helm, 1987), pp.51–75, quoted at p.51.
84. For a fuller account of Jacobs, Hamilton and other women physicians involved in peace activities at this time, see N. Lewer and P. van den Dungen, 'Women Physicians and Peace', in T.M. Ruprecht, C. Jenssen (eds), *Äskulap oder Mars?: Ärzte Gegen den Krieg* (Bremen: Donat Verlag, 1991).
85. H. Josephson (ed.), op. cit., p.379.
86. A. Wiltsher, *Most Dangerous Women: Feminist Peace Campaigners of the Great War* (London: Pandora, 1985), pp.103–25.
87. C. Benedict, 'Now I Dare Do It', in B. Cook (ed.), *Toward The Great Change* (New York: Garland Library of War and Peace, Garland Pub., 1976), pp.217–19.
88. R. Young (ed.), *Why Wars Must Cease* (New York: Macmillan, 1935).
89. H. Josephson (ed.), op. cit., p.380.
90. O. Nathan and H. Norden, *Einstein on Peace* (New York: Shocken Books, 1968), p.3.
91. This was smuggled out of Germany and published in Switzerland, in German, in 1917 as *Die Biologie des Krieges*. The English translation was published as *The Biology of War* (London: J.M. Dent, 1919).
92. W. Zuelzer, 'George Friedrich Nicolai', in *World Encyclopedia of Peace: Vol. 2* (Oxford: Pergamon Press, 1986), pp.42–5 Also see W. Zuelzer, *The Nicolai Case: A Biography* (Detroit: Wayne State University Press, 1982).
93. The three main intellectual inputs of Social Darwinism were racialism, selectionism and instinctivism. The use of Darwin's *Origin of the Species* (1859) in this context was unfortunate since Darwin did not view species and animals in terms of 'higher' and 'lower'. The apologists' thinking relates more to that of H. Spencer and his work *Descriptive Sociology*, written between 1873 and 1881. He saw evolution as a progression from simplicity to complexity, resulting in Man, the 'apotheosis of the evolutionary climb'. This anomaly is discussed in J. Burry, 'Social Spencerism is not Social Darwinism', *Medicine and War*, Vol. 5, No. 3, 1989, pp.148–50; and M. Ruse, *Taking Darwin Seriously: A naturalistic approach to philosophy* (New York: Blackwell, 1986).
94. B.W. Ike, 'From the Apologetics of War to Global Individualism', *Medicine and War*, Vol. 5, No. 1, 1989, pp.16–28.

95. Ibid., p. 21.
96. B. W. Ike, 'On "The Biology of War"', *Medicine and War*, Vol. 3, No. 1, 1987, pp. 33–42.
97. Ibid., p. 35.
98. D. Holdstock, 'Wilfred Trotter and the Biosociology of Peace and War', *Medicine and War*, Vol. 2, No. 1, 1986, pp. 43–50.
99. W. Trotter, *Instincts of the Herd in Peace and War* (London: Benn, 1916). The book was based on two papers published in 1908 and 1909 in *Sociological Review*, written shortly after his meeting with Freud in Vienna.
100. W. Trotter, *Instincts of the Herd in Peace and War* (London: Benn, 1940), twelfth impression, p. 17.
101. D. Holdstock, op. cit., p. 44.
102. In Pelican Freud Library, Vol. 12, *Civilisation, Society and Religion* (England: Penguin Books, 1985), pp. 61–76.
103. Ibid., p. 62.
104. Ibid., p. 72.
105. J. MacCurdy, *The Psychology of War* (London: Heinemann, 1918), pp. 51–2.
106. A. C. F. Beales, op. cit., p. 309.

PART THREE

1. R. C. Birch, *Britain and Europe, 1871–1939* (Oxford: Pergamon Press, 1966), p. 157.
2. Ibid., p. 194.
3. Ibid., p. 234.
4. S. J. Woolf (ed.), *European Fascism* (London: Weidenfeld & Nicolson, 1968), p. 23.
5. Ibid., p. 24.
6. R. C. Birch, op. cit., p. 162.
7. A. C. F. Beales, op. cit., p. 317.
8. M. Ceadel, 'The Peace Movement between the wars: problems of definition', in R. Taylor and N. Young (eds), op. cit., pp. 73–99.
9. Ibid., p. 91.
10. From War Resisters International, *Resistance and Reconstruction* (Gujarat, India: Institute for Total Revolution, 1988), p. 199. Also see H. R. Brown, *Cutting Ice* (Middlesex, England: War Resisters International, 1930).
11. B. de Ligt, *The Conquest of Violence* (London: George Routledge, 1937), pp. 269–85.
12. See the introduciton by Peter van den Dungen in the 1989 reprint of *The Conquest of Violence* (London: Pluto Press, 1989).
13. Reproduced in Netherlands Medical Association, *Medical Opinions on War* (Amsterdam: Elsevier, 1938), pp. 70–2.
14. B. W. Ike, 'Prevention of War in Medical Literature', *Current Research on Peace and Violence*, Vol. VII, No. 1, 1984, pp. 65–77.
15. See n. 13.
16. R. Thompson, 'The War Problem. A Psychological Approach', in Netherlands Medical Association, op. cit., pp. 11–14.
17. R. MacDonald Ladell, 'Imagination and War Prophylaxis', in Netherlands Medical

Association, op. cit., pp. 23–6.
18. L. Browne, 'Psychology and Peace', in Netherlands Medical Association, op. cit., pp. 15–22.
19. *The Lancet,* 22 August 1936, p. 465. The letter was signed by MPC's secretary, Cecile Booysen.
20. *The Lancet,* 26 September 1936, p. 761. See also *World Peace Congress Brussels, 3–6 September 1936* (Brussels: 'Labor', 1936), pp. 136–8.
21. Published in English as *Why War? Open letters between Einstein and Freud* (London: The New Commonwealth [A Society for the Promotion of International Law and Order], 1934).
22. A useful discussion on this is found in N. J. Lavik, 'Contributions from Psychiatry on the Peace–War Issue', *Bulletin of Peace Proposals,* Vol. 20, No. 2, 1989, pp. 157–65.
23. R. Britton, *What Influences Us to Accept War?* Paper read at Medical Association for the Prevention of War conference on 'The Right to Wage War', 11 May 1985, London.
24. H. Joules (ed.), *The Doctor's View on War* (Woking: Unwin Bros., 1938).
25. Ibid., p. 102. (Chapter 9 was entitled 'Doctors and the State'. The author of the chapter is not given but contributors to the book are listed as Drs H. Joules, Mary Day, T. A. Ross, P. A. Gorer, R. R. Bomford, T. D. Day, W. Howard Hughes and Prof. W. H. Wynn.)
26. Ibid., p. 106. See also a letter in *The Lancet,* 4 December 1937, from Somerville Hastings.
27. *The Lancet,* 23 July 1938, p. 206.
28. *Peace News,* 9 January 1937, p. 9.
29. The article, see n. 28, gave no further details about the pamphlet.
30. *The Lancet,* 'Preparation for Air-Raids', 5 December 1936, p. 1340. This was compiled from a meeting, organised by the MPC, at BMA House, to discuss protection for civilians against aerial attack, particularly in working class areas.
31. Cambridge Scientists Anti-War Group, *Protection of the Public from Aerial Attack* (London: Victor Gollancz, 1937). Reviews of this can be found in *Peace News* of 27 February 1937, p. 9, and 31 July 1937, p. 5.
32. *The Lancet,* 26 June 1937, p. 1542.
33. J. Athey, 'Karel Capek's New Peace Play', *Peace News,* 27 February 1937, p. 9.
34. C. L. Mowat, *Britain Between The Wars: 1918–1945* (London: Methuen, 1968), p. 538.
35. H. R. L. Sheppard, *We Say No* (London: John Murray, 1935), p. 142.
36. H. Josephson (ed.), op. cit., pp. 652–4.
37. R. Rusk and J. Scotland, *Doctrines of the Great Educators* (London: Macmillan Education, 1979), 5th ed., p. 196.
38. M. Remiddi, 'Maria Montessori: A Vision of Man Transformed', *UNESCO Courier,* Vol. 17, April 1964, p. 19.
39. Ibid., p. 20.
40. H. Josephson (ed.), op. cit., p. 653.
41. B. de Ligt, op. cit., p. 215.
42. Ibid., Appendix 1, p. 286. The method which Montessori refers to in the first paragraph of the quote is the non-violent direct action approach to the opposition of war as proposed by de Ligt and others in WRI. For example see p. 34 of n. 11.
43. H. Josephson (ed.), op. cit., p. 653.
44. Y. Sandoz, 'The Red Cross and Peace: Realities and Limits', *Journal of Peace*

Research, Vol. 24, No. 3, 1987.
45. *The Lancet*, 8 January 1938, pp. 90–1.
46. Ibid.
47. Personal communication: 10 April 1988.

PART FOUR

1. N. Young, 'Tradition and innovation in the British Peace Movement: towards an analytical framework', in R. Taylor and N. Young (eds), *Campaign for Peace* (Manchester: Manchester University Press, 1987), p. 10.
2. L.S. Wittner, 'The Transnational Movement against Nuclear Weapons, 1945–1986: A Preliminary Survey', in C. Chatfield and P. Van Den Dungen (eds), *Peace Movements and Political Cultures* (Knoxville: University of Tennessee Press, 1988).
3. B.W. Ike, 'Prevention of War in Medical Literature', *Current Research on Peace and Violence*, Vol. VII, No. 1, 1984.
4. P.P. Everts, 'The Peace Movement and Public Opinion: Prospects for theNineties', paper presented at the 30th Annual Convention of the International Studies Association, London, March 1989.
5. Wittner, op. cit., p. 169.
6. R. Doll, H. Joules, L. Penrose, et al., *The Lancet*, 20 January 1951, p. 170.
7. D. Sheldon, *The Lancet*, 27 January 1951, p. 235.
8. Bohemicus, *The Lancet*, 27 January 1951, p. 235.
9. M. McCauley, *The Origins of the Cold War* (London: Longman, 1983).
10. M. Penrose, 'Anti-war medics fight on', *General Practitioner*, 13 March 1981.
11. Reported in *MAPW Bulletin No. 1*, May 1951.
12. Reported in *MAPW Bulletin No. 2*, July 1951.
13. *The Lancet*, 10 May 1958, p. 1028.
14. Personal communication. 22 January 1990. According to one senior member of the Association des Médecins Français pour la Prévention de la Guerre Nucléaire (AMFPGN) 'the whole affair was hushed up ... as usually happens over here [France]'.
15. K. Arnung, personal communication, February 1990.
16. Reported in *MAPW Bulletin*, November 1951.
17. H. Vickers, letter in *British Medical Journal*, 4 August 1951, pp. 300–1.
18. D. Leys and L. Penrose, letter in *British Medical Journal*, 11 August 1951, p. 363.
19. H. Vickers, op. cit.
20. C. Watney-Roe, letter in *British Medical Journal*, 11 September 1951, p. 102.
21. Letter dated 9 March 1953 from L.S. Penrose (MAPW Hon. Sec.) to Morgan Phillips (Sec. Labour Party). In MAPW archives.
22. Letter dated 2 July 1953 from Morgan Phillips to L.S. Penrose. In MAPW archives.
23. Letter to Morgan Phillips from MAPW, dated 10 June 1953. In MAPW archives.
24. Lionel S.Penrose (1898–1972), Obituary in *Proceedings of MAPW*, Vol. 2, Part 5 (1972), pp. 117–22. A collection of Penrose's papers are lodged at University College, London. See M. Merrington, B. Blundell et al., *A list of the papers and correspondence of Lionel Sharples Penrose* (Publications Office, University College London, 1979).

Notes

25. J. Segall, 'Establishing Peace', Editorial in *Medicine and War*, Vol. 5, No. 1, 1989, pp. 1–4.
26. L. Penrose, *On the Objective Study of Crowd Behaviour* (London: H.K. Lewis & Co., 1952), p. 68. A useful discussion of Penrose's ideas may be found in *The Lancet*, 9 February 1952, pp. 300–1.
27. Penrose obituary, op. cit., p. 120.
28. M. Penrose, 'Three Decades of MAPW', *Proceedings of MAPW*, Vol. 3, Part 4 (March 1980), pp. 125–8.
29. 'The Bombs', editorial in *The Lancet*, 17 April 1954, p. 815.
30. *The Times*, 7 March 1954.
31. A. Comfort, letter in *The Lancet*, 24 April 1954, p. 887.
32. D. Stafford-Clark, letter in *The Lancet*, 1 May 1954.
33. H. Josephson (ed.), op. cit., pp. 860–2.
34. A. Schweitzer, *The Problem of Peace in the World of Today. Nobel Peace Prize Address* (London: Adam & Charles Black, 1954), p. 20.
35. A. Schweitzer, *Peace or Atomic War? (Three broadcast appeals from Oslo on 28/29/30 April 1958)* (London: Adam & Charles Black, 1958).
36. H. Josephson, op. cit., p. 862.
37. J. Rotblat, 'The Pugwash Conferences on Science and World Affairs', *Medicine and War*, Vol. 1, No. 1, 1985, pp. 51–4.
    J. Rotblat, *Pugwash – The First Ten Years* (New York: Humanities Press, 1968).
38. J. Rotblat, *History of the Pugwash Conferences* (London: Taylor & Francis, 1962).
39. H. Josephson (ed.), op. cit., pp. 306–7.
40. E. Fromm, *The Sane Society* (New York: Holt, Rinehart and Winston, 1955).
41. E. Fromm, 'Indifference to Life', in D. Roussopoulos (ed.), *Our Generation Against Nuclear War* (Montreal: Black Rose Books, 1985), pp. 409–11.
42. L.S. Wittner, op. cit., p. 270.
43. J. Minnion, P. Bolsover (eds), *The CND Story* (London: Allison and Busby, 1983). See also C. Driver, *The Disarmers: A Study in Protest* (London: Hodder & Stoughton, 1964).
44. Personal communication, 15 March 1988.
45. The committee consisted of Drs David Nathan, H. Jack Geiger, and Victor Sidel – all at Harvard Medical School – and Bernard Lown, then at the Harvard School of Public Health.
46. V. Sidel, J. Geiger, B. Lown et al., 'The Medical Consequences of Thermonuclear War', *New England Journal of Medicine*, Vol. 255, 31 May 1962, pp. 1126–55.
47. Ibid., p. 1126.
48. US Congress Joint Committeee on Atomic Energy, *Biological and Environmental Effects of Nuclear War* (1959).
49. A report in 1962, the 'Baby Tooth Survey', by paediatrician Albert Schwartz in St. Louis, clearly demonstrated a major increase in Strontium 90 in children's first teeth between 1950 and 1954. The report was sponsored by the Committee for Nuclear Information, St. Louis. See also Medical Research Council, 'Radioactive fall-out and the testing of Nuclear Weapons', *Nature*, Vol. 192 (1962), pp. 400–3.
50. S. Aranow, F. Erwin and V. Sidel (eds), *The Fallen Sky: Medical Consequences of Thermonuclear War* (Hill & Wang, 1963).
51. PSR, *PSR Rx: The Only Cure for Nuclear War is Prevention* (Washington: PSR, n.d.).
52. P. Boyer, 'From Activism to Apathy. The American People and Nuclear Weapons,

1963–1980', *Journal of American History*, Vol. 70, March 1984, pp. 821–44.
53. J. Brown, ' "A is for Atom, B is for Bomb"; Civil Defence in American Public Education, 1948–1963', *Journal of American History*, Vol. 75, No. 1, June 1988, pp. 68–90.
54. For example, the proceedings of an MAPW conference held in Oxford 1962, were published as *The Pathogenesis of War* (London: Lewis, 1963).
The Times Literary Supplement, 19 July 1963, called the book a 'group of intelligent and coherent essays' ... 'hoping that MAPW meembers will not overlook the problem of getting their sane views heard and seeing that some steps are taken to give practical effect to their suggestions'.
55. B.W. Ike (1984), op. cit., p. 67.
56. For her biography see Helen Caldicott, *Current Biography*, October 1983, pp. 9–13.
57. H. Caldicott, *Nuclear Madness: What you can Do!* (London: Wildwood House, 1978).
58. Then Assistant Minister of Heath, Chazov was probably the foremost researcher in cardiology in the USSR. He later became Minister of Health and a Politburo member.
59. B. Day and H. Waitzkin, 'The Medical Profession and Nuclear War', *Journal of American Medical Association*, Vol. 254, No. 5, 1985, pp. 644–51.
60. A detailed account of this meeting is given in G. Warner and M. Shuman, *Citizen Diplomats* (New York: Continuum Press, 1987), Ch. 1.
61. *IPPNW – Description and Brief History* (Boston: IPPNW, September 1986), p. 4.
62. J. Humphrey, 'The Development of the Physicians, Movements', *Medicine and War*, Vol. 1, No. 2, 1985, pp. 87–99.
63. Official Statement by the Norwegian Nobel Committee, 11 October 1985.
64. *The Daily Express*, Editorial, 12 December 1985.
65. Editorial, 'A Re-Awakening', *Proceedings of MAPW*, Vol. 3, Part 5 (March 1981), pp. 155–6.
66. J. Humphrey, op. cit., p. 92.
67. C. Gray and K. Payne, 'Victory is Possible', *Foreign Policy*, No. 39, Summer 1980, pp. 14–27.
68. P. Webber, G. Wilkinson, B. Rubin, *Crisis Over Cruise: A Plain Guide to the New Weapons* (London: Penguin Books, 1983).
69. Quote from US Admiral Gene LaRoque, *New Statesman*, 31 October 1981.
70. J. Garrison and P. Shivpuri, *The Russian Threat* (London: Gateway Books, 1983), p. 24.
71. *Protect and Survive* (London: HMSO, 1980).
72. Editorial, 'Threat of Nuclear War', *The Lancet*, 15 November 1980, p. 1061.
73. *The Preparation and Organisation of the Health Services for War. Home Defence Circular (77)* (London: DHSS, 1977).
74. F. Brockway, 'World Disarmament Campaign', *Journal of MAPW*, Vol. 3, Part 9 June 1983, pp. 414–16, and *Disarmament Fact Sheet No. 26* (New York: Department for Disarmament Affairs, United Nations, December 1982).
75. British Medical Association: Board of Science and Education, *The Medical Effects of Nuclear War* (London: John Wiley & Sons for the BMA, 1983). Annex 6 of the report looked in detail at HDC(77)1 and its associated memoranda eg., ES10/1974: Survival Under Fallout Conditions.
76. Quoted in D. Josephs, '1983–1988. The BMA and the Nuclear Issue', *Medicine and War*, Vol. 5, No. 3, 1989, pp. 137–47.

Notes

77. Ibid., p. 140.
78. S. Watkins, *Medicine and Labour: The Politics of a Profession* (London: Lawrence & Wishart, 1987).
79. Ibid., p. 200.
80. D. Josephs, op. cit., p. 141.
81. *Effects of nuclear war on health and health services: Report of the international committee of experts in medical sciences and public health* (Geneva: WHO, March 1984; second edition 1987).
82. *The Guardian*, 3 March 1984.
83. See n. 46.
84. B.W. Ike, op. cit., p. 69.
85. S. Roth, 'Civil Defence in the USA', *Medicine and War*, Vol. 1, No. 2, 1985, pp. 119–23.
86. J. Leaning and L. Keyes (eds), *The Counterfeit Arc: Crisis Relocation for Nuclear War* (Massachusetts: Bollinger Pub. Co., 1983).
87. See n. 59.
88. Study Group: Faculty of Community Medicine, 'Implications of nuclear weapons for community medicine', *Community Medicine*, Vol. 4, 1982, pp. 34–9.
89. Central Office of Information, *Civil Protection Planning for Major Emergencies at a National and Local Level* (London: HMSO, 1986).
90. Particularly HDC(77)1; HM(85)16; and HC(88)31, which were circulated by the DHSS.
91. G. Kersley, 'Civil Defence in a Nuclear Disaster', *Medicine and War*, Vol. 1, No. 2, 1985, pp. 109–14.
92. A. Haines, 'The Role of Civil Defence in a Nuclear War', *Proceedings of MAPW*, Vol. 3, Part 7 (1982), pp. 275–93.
    P. Sepping, 'Civil Defence in the UK', *Medicine and War*, Vol. 1, No. 2, 1985, pp. 115–18.
    P. Sims, 'A Dilemma for Doctors', *Medicine and War*, Vol. 2, No. 3, 1986, pp. 199–200.
93. M. Howard, 'Reviving Civil Defence', *The Times*, 30 January 1980.
94. E.P. Thompson, *Protest and Survive* (Nottingham: Russell Press Ltd., 1980).
95. See n. 71.
96. See n. 91.
97. D. Hencke, 'How to survive the bomb and save on overheads', The Guardian, 11 October 1983.
98. See n. 96.
99. Faculty of Community Medicine of the Royal Colleges of Physicians of the United Kingdom, *The Role of the Community Physician in the Promotion of Peaceful International Relations and in the Prevention of War* (June 1988).
100. *Health for all by the year 2000: Charter for Action* (Faculty of Community Medicine, 1986).
101. See n. 81.
102. C. Ryle and J. Garrison, *Citizen Diplomacy* (London: Merlin Press, 1986).
     N. Lewer, 'Mediation: Developing a New Role for Physicians in Peacemaking Processes', *Medicine and War*, Vol. 6, No. 1 (1990), pp. 33–6.
103. See n. 96.
104. S. Hadjipavalou and G. Carr-Hill, 'A Revised Set of Blast Casualty Rates for Civil Defence Use: An Overview', *Journal of Royal Statistical Society Association*, Vol. 152, 1989, pp. 157–68.

105. S. Openshaw, et al., *Doomsday: Britain after Nuclear Attack* (Oxford: Blackwell, 1983).
106. Office of Technology Assessment, *The Effects of Nuclear War* (London: Croom Helm, 1980).
107. D. Holdstock, 'The Home Office and Nuclear Weapons Effects: A Small Step in the Right Direction', *Medicine and War*, Vol. 5, No. 2, 1989, pp. 67–8.
108. See n. 89.
109. R. P. Turco, O. B. Toon, et al., 'Nuclear Winter: Global Consequences of Multiple Nuclear Explosions', *Science*, Vol. 22, 1983, pp. 1283–92.
110. L. Dotto, *Planet Earth in Jeopardy* (Chichester: John Wiley, 1983). This is a condensed version of the lengthy SCOPE-ENUWAR Reports.
111. British Medical Association, *Selection of Casualties for Treatment after Nuclear Attack*, Report of the Board of Science and Education (BMA, 1988).
112. See n. 75.
113. J. Leaning, 'Physicians, Triage and Nuclear War', *The Lancet*, 30 July 1988, p. 269.
114. *MCANW Newsletters No. 23*, MCANW, London, Winter 1988.
115. A. Haines, C. de B White, and J. Gleisner, 'Nuclear Weapons and Medicine: Some Ethical Dilemmas', *Journal of Medical Ethics*, Vol. 9, Part 4, 1983, pp. 200–6.
116. See Part Three, n. 24.
117. J. A. Verdoorn, *Mars en Aesculapius* (Lochem, Holland: De Tijdstroom, 1985). These notes are taken directly from a review of the book by S. Tillema, in *Medicine and War*, Vol. 2, No. 1, 1986, pp. 65–6.
118. C. Cassel, et al., 'The Physician's Oath and the Prevention of Nuclear War', *Medicine and War*, Vol. 2, No. 1, 1986, pp. 51–6.
119. D. Krech, 'The Challenge and the Promise', *Journal of Social Issues*, Vol. 2, 1946, pp. 2–6. This article was a report from the short-lived Committee of International Peace which had been set up by the Society for the Psychological Study of Social Issues (SPSSI) in the US, 1945.
120. J. Morawski and S. Goldstein, 'Psychology and Nuclear War. A Chapter in Our Legacy of Social Responsibility', *American Psychologist*, March 1985, pp. 276–84.
121. J. D. Frank, 'Breaking Through the Barrier: Psychological Challenges in the Nuclear Age', *Psychiatry*, Vol. 23, 1960, pp. 245–66.
    J. D. Frank, 'Emotional and Motivational Aspects of the Disarmament Problem', *Journal of Social Issues*, Vol. 17, No. 3, 1961, pp. 20–27.
    J. D. Frank, *Sanity and Survival* (New York: Random House, 1967).
122. R. J. Lifton, *Death in Life* (New York: Random House, 1968).
    R. J. Lifton, 'Beyond Psychic Numbing: A Call to Awareness', *American Journal of Orthopsychiatry*, Vol. 52, No. 4, 1982, pp. 619–29.
123. J. E. Mack, 'Psychosocial Effects of the Nuclear Arms Race', *Bulletin of the Atomic Scientists*, Vol. 37, No. 4, 1981, pp. 18–23.
124. R. Holt, 'Can Psychology Meet Einstein's Challenge?' *Political Psychology*, Vol. 5, No. 2, 1984, pp. 199–224.
125. Quoted in O. and H. Norden, op. cit., p. 376.
126. A. d'Heurle, 'The Role of Psychology in the Development of the Theories and Strategies of Peace', *Current Reseearch on Peace and Violence*, Vol. X, No. 2–3, 1987, pp. 71–7.
127. N. Lavik, 'Contributions from Psychiatry on the Peace–War Issue', *Bulletin of Peace Proposals*, Vol. 20, No. 2, 1989, pp. 157–65.

128. M. Deutsch, 'The Prevention of World War III. A Psychological Perspective', *Political Psychology*, Vol. 4, 1983, pp. 3–32.
129. Themes of these congresses have included; Nuclear Illusions – The Human Cost; Co-Operation not Confrontation; and Maintain Life on Earth.
130. D. B. Menkes, 'Psychological Defence Mechanisms and the Nuclear Arms Race: An Interactive Model', *Medicine and War*, Vol. 5, No. 2, 1989, pp. 80–95.
131. In a paper given at the 2nd IPPNW World Congress, Cambridge, UK, 3–7 April 1982.
132. U. Bronfenbrenner, 'The Mirror-image in Soviet-American Relations: A social Psychologist's report', *Journal of Social Issues*, Vol. 17, No. 3, 1961, pp. 45–56.
133. J. Thompson, 'Tribalism and the Arms Race Trap', *Medicine and War*, Vol. 4, No. 1, 1988, pp. 37–47.
134. E. H. Erikson, 'Pseudospeciation in the Nuclear Age', *Political Psychology*, Vol. 6, No. 2, 1985, pp. 213–17.
135. D. Ingleby, 'Limitations of the Psychological Approach to War and Peace', *Current Research on Peace and Violence*, Vol. X, No. 2–3, 1987, pp. 78–82.
136. Also see A. Eskola, 'Can Social-Psychology Contribute to Peacemaking and Peacebuilding?' *Current Research on Peace and Violence*, Vol. X, No. 2–3, 1987, pp. 66–70.
137. L. Doob, 'A Cyprus Workshop: An Exercise in Intervention Methodology. *Journal of Social Psychology*, Vol. 94, 1974, pp. 161–78.
138. H. Kelman, 'The Problem-Solving Workshop: A Social Psychological Contribution to the Resolution of International Conflicts', *Journal of Peace Research*, Vol. XIII, No. 2, 1976, pp. 79–90.
139. J. Burton, *Resolving Deep-Rooted Conflict: A Handbook* (New York: University Press of America, 1987).
140. One definition of *Mediation* is: a process which aims to remove psychological obstacles such as misperceptions, prejudices and irrational fears that prevent people in conflict meeting for constructive talks. This may be facilitated by an impartial third party, the *mediator*.
See A. Curle, *In the Middle: Non-Official Mediation in Violence Situations* (Leamington Spa: Berg Pubs., 1986).

CONCLUSION

1. C. Legum, 'Amin is syphilis victim, his former doctor says', *Washington Post*, 30 April 1977.
2. J. Humphrey, 'Some Personal Reflections', *The Lancet*, 12 December 1987, pp. 1389–90.
3. M. Nusbaumer and J. DiLorio, 'The Medicalisation of Nuclear Disarmament Claims', *Peace and Change*, Vol. XI, No. 1, Spring 1985, pp. 63–73.
4. 'MAPW Written Statement to UNSSD2: The two main proposals', *Journal of the Medical Association for the Prevention of War*, Vol. 3, Part 8, Autumn 1982, pp. 382–5; and, 'Network for a UN Second Assembly', *Journal of the Medical Association for the Prevention of War*, Vol. 3, Part 12, October 1984, pp. 730–2.
5. INFUSA Briefing Paper. *Conferences on a UN Organised Democratically (UNODEM) for World Peace and Justice*, December 1989.

6. L. Sivard, *World Military and Social Expenditures 1989* (Washington: World Priorities, 1989).
7. I. Munro, 'IPPNW in a changing world', *The Lancet*, Vol. 336, 29 September 1990, pp. 802–4.
8. IPPNW Information Leaflet, *IPPNW Programs for 1990*.
9. P. Zheutlin, 'Doctors join GE boycott', *The Bulletin of Atomic Scientists*, November 1990, p. 8.
10. Ibid.
11. F. Castillo, 'The International Physicians for the Prevention of Nuclear War: Transnational Midwife of World Peace', *Medicine and War*, Vol. 6, No. 4, 1990, pp. 250–68.
12. Also similar foundations in other countries, such as Rehabilitation Centre for Torture Victims (RCT) in Denmark; see O. V. Rasmussen, 'Medical Aspects of Torture', *Medicine and War*, Vol. 6, No. 4, 1990, pp. 299–309; and T. W. Harding, 'Prevention of Torture and Inhuman or Degrading Treatment: Medical Implications of a New European Convention', *The Lancet*, 27 May 1989, pp. 1191–3.
13. Information pamphlet issued by Medical Group of Amnesty International in the UK.
14. Also see 'Sudan: Repression of Doctors', *The Lancet*, 24 November 1990, pp. 1307–8.
15. *The Berlin Declaration of European Leaders of the International Physicians for the Prevention of Nuclear War* (Berlin, 14 January 1990).

BIBLIOGRAPHY

Adams, R. and Cullen, S. *The Final Epidemic: Physicians and Scientists on Nuclear War*, Educational Foundation for Nuclear Science, Chicago, US, 1981.
Allen, D. *The Fight for Peace, Vol. 1.* Garland Publishing Inc., New York, 1971.
Aranow, S., Erwin, F., Sidel, V. (eds.). *The Fallen Sky: Medical Consequences of Thermonuclear War*, Hill & Wang, New York, 1963.
Association Médicale Internationale contre la Guerre. *Actes & Manifestations Diverses (1905–1910)*, Bouchy & Co., Paris, 1910.
Avery, J., *Health Effects of War and the Threat of War: An introduction to the literature.* WHO Regional Office for Europe, Copenhagen, 1988.
Baccino-Astrada, A. *Manual on the Rights and Duties of Medical Personnel in Armed Conflicts*, ICRC, Geneva, 1982.
Barnett, L. and Lee, I. (eds.). *The Nuclear Mentality – A Psychosocial Analysis of the Arms Race.* MCANW/Pluto, London, 1989.
Beales, A.C.F. *The History of Peace*, G. Bell & Sons, London, 1931.
Beaumont, B. 'Medical Care: The Nuclear Aftermath', *Proceedings of MAPW*, Vol. 3, Part 7, 1982, pp. 294–305.
Beer, F.A., *Peace Against War: The Ecology of International Violence*, W.H. Freeman & Co., San Francisco, 1981.
Benedict, C. 'Now I Dare Do It', in Cook, B. (ed.), *Toward the Great Change*, Garland Library of War and Peace, Garland Pubs., New York, 1976.
Birch, R.C. *Britain and Europe 1871–1939*, Pergamon Press Ltd., London, 1966.
Boxer, M.A. 'Socialism Faces Feminism', in Boxer, M.A. and Quataert, J.H., *Socialist Women*, New York, 1978.
Boyer, P. 'From Activism to Apathy. The American People and Nuclear Weapons, 1963–1980', *Journal of American History*, Vol. 70, March 1984, pp. 821–44.
Boyer, P. 'Physicians Confront the Apocalypse: The American Medical Profession and the Threat of Nuclear War', *Journal of American Medical Association*, Vol. 254, 1985, pp. 633–43.
Bradley, D. *No Place To Hide*, Little, Brown & Company, Boston, 1948.
British Medical Association. *The Handbook of Medical Ethics*, British Medical Association, London, 1981.
British Medical Association: Board of Science and Education. *The Medical Effects of Nuclear War*, John Wiley & Sons, London, 1983.
British Medical Association: Board of Science and Education. *Selection of Casualties for Treatment after Nuclear Attack*, BMA, London, 1988.
Brittain, V. *The Rebel Passion: A Short History of Some Pioneer Peacemakers*, George Allen & Unwin Ltd., London, 1964.
Brock, P. *Pacifism in Europe to 1914*, Princeton University Press, US, 1972.
Brockway, F. 'World Disarmament Campaign', *Journal of Medical Association for the Prevention of War*, Vol. 3, Part 9, June 1983, pp. 414–16.
Bronfenbrenner, U. 'The Mirror-image in Soviet–American Relations: A Social Psycho-

logist's Report', *Journal of Social Issues*, Vol. 17, No. 3, 1961, pp. 45–56.
Brown, J. ' "A is for Atom, B is for Bomb": Civil Defense in American Public Education, 1948–1963', *Journal of American History*, Vol. 75, No. 1, 1988, pp. 69–90.
Bruwer, A. 'Nuclear War, Patriotism, and Medical Ethics', *The Pharos*, Summer 1982, pp. 2–8.
Burry, J. 'Social Spenserism not Social Darwinism', *Medicine and War*, Vol. 5, No. 3, 1989, pp. 148–50.
Buttery, C.M.G. 'The Physician and Radiation Fallout', *Virginia Medical Monthly*, Vol. 90, 1963, pp. 567–72.
Caldicott, H. *Nuclear Madness: What you can do!*, Wildwood House, London, 1978.
Cambridge Scientists Anti-War Group. *Protection of the Public from Aerial Attack*, Victor Gollancz, London, 1937.
Carver, Lord. 'Morale in Battle – The Medical and the Military', *Journal of the Royal Society of Medicine*, Vol. 82, Feb. 1989, pp. 67–71.
Cassel, C. et al., 'The Physician's Oath and the Prevention of Nuclear War', *Medicine and War*, Vol. 2, No. 1, 1986, pp. 51–6.
Cassel, C. and Jameton, A.J. 'Medical Responsibility and Thermonuclear War', *Annals of Internal Medicine*, Vol. 97, 1982, pp. 426–32.
Castillo, F. 'The International Physicians for the Prevention of Nuclear War: Transnational Midwife of World Peace', *Medicine and War*, Vol. 6, No. 4, 1990, pp. 250–68.
Central Office of Information. *Civil Protection: Planning for Major Emergencies at a National and Local Level*, HMSO, London, 1986.
Chatfield, C. (ed.), *Peace Movements in America*, Shocken Books, New York, 1973.
Chazov, I., Ilyin, L., Guskova, A. *The Danger of Nuclear War: Soviet Physicians' Perspective*, Novosti Press Agency Publishing House, Moscow, 1982.
Childress, J.F. 'Citizen and Physician: Harmonius or Conflicting Responsibilities?', *Journal of Medicine and Philosophy*, Vol. 2, No. 4, 1977, pp. 401–9.
Chisholm, B. *Prescriptions for Survival*, Columbia University Press, New York, US, 1957.
Chivian, E., Chivian, S., Lifton, R.J., Mack, J. (eds.). *Last Aid: The Medical Dimensions of Nuclear War*, W.H. Freeman, San Francisco, 1982.
Cooper, S.E. 'Women's Participation in European Peace Movements. The Struggle to Prevent WW1', in Pierson, R.R. (ed.) *Women and Peace. Theoretical, Historical and Practical Perspectives*, Croom Helm, London, 1987.
Day, B. and Waitzkin, H. 'The Medical Profession and Nuclear War', *Journal of American Medical Association*, Vol. 254, No. 5, 1985, pp. 644–51.
Dotto, L., *Planet Earth in Jeopardy*, John Wiley, Chichester, 1983.
Driver, C. *The Disarmers: A Study in Protest*, Hodder & Stoughton, London, 1964.
Durbin, E. and Bowlby, J. *Personal Aggressiveness and War*. Routledge & Kegan Paul, London, 1939.
Eisenberg, L. 'Virchow: Physician as Politician', *Medicine and War*, Vol. 2, No. 4, 1986, pp. 243–50.
Ellis, Havelock. *The Philosophy of Conflict, and other Essays in War Time. Second Series*, Constable & Co., London, 1918.
Erikson, E.H. 'Pseudospeciation in the Nuclear Age', *Political Psychology*, Vol. 6, No. 2, 1985, pp. 213–17.
Eskola, A. 'Can Social-Psychology Contribute to Peacemaking and Peacebuilding?', *Current Research on Peace and Violence*, Vol. X, No. 2–3, 1987, pp. 66–70.
Faculty of Community Medicine of Royal College of Physicians, UK. *The Role of the*

Community Physician in the Promotion of Peaceful International Relations and in the Prevention of War, June 1988.
Fenton, I. (ed.) The Psychology of Nuclear Conflict, Coventure Ltd., London, 1986.
Fischoff, A. 'On The Reduction of Continental Armies', in Cooper, S. (ed.), Arms Limitations, Garland Library of War and Peace, New York, 1972.
Forsythe, D. 'Humanitarian Mediation by the International Committee of the Red Cross', in Touval, S. and Zartman, W. (eds.), International Mediation in Theory and Practice, Westview Press, Colorado, 1985, pp. 233–49.
Frank, J.D. 'Breaking through the Barrier: Psychological Challenges in the Nuclear Age', Psychiatry, Vol. 23, No. 3, 1960, pp. 245–66.
Frank, J.D. 'Emotional and Motivational Aspects of the Disarmament Problem', Journal of Social Issues, Vol. 17, No. 3, 1961, pp. 20–7.
Frank, J.D. Sanity and Survival: Psychological Aspects of War and Peace, Random House, New York, 1967.
Fried, A. Handbuch der Friedensbewegung. Zweiter Teil, Verlag der 'Friedens-Warte', Berlin and Leipzig, 1913.
Fromm, E. The Sane Society, Holt, Rinehart & Winston, New York, 1955.
Fromm, E. 'Indifference to Life', in Roussopoulos, D. (ed.), Our Generation Against Nuclear War, Black Rose Books, Montreal, 1985, pp. 409–11.
Garraty, J., Sternstein, J. (eds.). Encyclopedia of American Biography, Harper & Row, New York, 1974.
Geiger, H.J. 'Hidden Professional Roles: The Physician as Reactionary', Social Policy, Vol. 1, No. 6, March/April 1974, pp. 24–33.
Gellert, G. 'Global Health Interdependence and the International Physicians' Movement', Journal of the American Medical Association, Vol. 264, No. 5, 1 August 1990, pp. 610–13.
Gigon, F. The Epic of The Red Cross, Jarrolds Ltd., London.
Glover, E. War, Sadism and Pacifism, Allen & Unwin, London, 1933.
Gray, C., Payne, K. 'Victory is Possible', Foreign Policy, No. 39, Summer 1980, pp. 14–27.
Grimes, F.M. Adventurers for Peace, Herbert Jones & Son, Nottingham, 1937.
Hadjipavalou, S., Carr-Hill, G. 'A Revised Set of Blast Casualty Rates for Civil Defense Use: An Overview', Journal of Royal Statistical Society Association, Vol. 152, 1989, pp. 157–68.
Haines, A. 'The Role of Civil Defense in Nuclear War', Proceedings of MAPW, Vol. 3, Part 7, 1982, pp. 275–93.
Haines, A., de B. White, C., Gleisner, J. 'Nuclear Weapons and Medicine: Some Ethical Dilemmas', Journal of Medical Ethics, Vol. 9, Part 4, 1983, pp. 200–6.
Harding, D.W. The Impulse to Dominate, George Allen & Unwin Ltd., London, 1941.
d'Heurle, A. 'The Role of Psychology in the Development of the Theories and Strategies of Peace', Current Research on Peace and Violence, Vol. X, No. 2–3, 1987, pp. 71–7.
Hinsley, F.H. Power and the Pursuit of Peace, Cambridge University Press, Cambridge, UK, 1963.
Holdstock, D. 'Wilfred Trotter and the Biosociology of Peace and War', Medicine and War, Vol. 2, No. 1, 1986, pp. 43–50.
Holdstock, D. 'The Home Office and Nuclear Weapons Effects: A Small Step in the Right Direction', Medicine and War, Vol. 5, No. 2, 1989, pp. 67–8.
Holdstock, D., 'Arms or Health: A Role for Medical Colleges?', Journal of the Royal College of Physicians of London, Vol. 23, No. 3, July 1989, pp. 185–8.

Holt, R. 'Can Psychology Meet Einstein's Challenge?', *Political Psychology*, Vol. 5, No. 2, 1984, pp. 199–224.
Howard, M. *War and the Liberal Conscience*, Oxford University Press, Oxford, 1981.
Humphrey, J. 'The Development of the Physicians' Peace Movements', *Medicine and War*, Vol. 1, No. 2, 1985, pp. 87–99.
Humphrey, J. 'Some Personal Reflections', *The Lancet*, 12 December 1987, pp. 1389–90.
ICRC. *The Geneva Conventions of August 12 1949*, ICRC, Geneva.
ICRC. *Protocols additional to the Geneva Conventions of 12 August 1949*, ICRC, Geneva, 1977.
ICRC. *To Promote Peace: Resolutions on Peace adopted by the International Movement of the Red Cross since 1921*, ICRC, Geneva, July 1986.
Ike, B. W. 'Prevention of War in Medical Literature, *Current Research on Peace and Violence*, Vol. VII, No. 1, 1984, pp. 65–77.
Ike, B. W. 'On "The Biology of War"', *Medicine and War*, Vol. 3, No. 1, 1987, pp. 33–42.
Ike, B. W., 'From the Apologetics of War to Global Individualism', *Medicine and War*, Vol. 5, No. 1, 1989, pp. 16–28.
Ingleby, D. 'Limitations on the Psychological Approach to War and Peace', *Current Research on Peace and Violence*, Vol. X, No. 2–3, 1987, pp. 78–82.
IPPNW. *Description and Brief History*, IPPNW, September, 1986.
Jonsen, A. R., Jameton, A. J. 'Social and Political Responsibilities of Physicians', *Journal of Medicine and Philosophy*, Vol. 2, 1977, pp. 376–400.
Jorge, R. *La Guerre et la Pensée Médicale*, Edition de la Societé des Sciences Médicales, Lisbon, Portugal, 1914.
Josephs, D. '1983 to 1988. The BMA and the Nuclear Issue', *Medicine and War*, Vol. 5, No. 3, 1989, pp. 137–47.
Josephs, D., Sims, P. 'War Planning in the Health Service – A Survey of Community Physicians', *Community Medicine*, Vol. 8, Part 1, 1986, pp. 58–71.
Josephson, H. (ed.). *Biographical Dictionary of Modern Peace Leaders*, Greenwood Press, London, 1984.
Joules, H. (ed.). *The Doctor's View on War*, Unwin Bros., Woking, 1938.
Kersley, G. 'Civil Defence in a Nuclear Disaster', *Medicine and War*, Vol. 1, No. 2, 1985, pp. 109–14.
Lambert, P. 'Benjamin Rush: Physicians in Politics', *Journal of Oklahoma State Medical Association*, Vol. 65, June 1972, pp. 218–24.
LaVigna, C. 'The Marxist Ambivalence Toward Women: Between Socialism and Feminism in the Italian Socialist Party', in Boxer, M. A. and Quataert, J. H., *Socialist Women*, New York, 1978.
Lavik, N. J. 'Contributions from Psychiatry on the Peace–War Issue', *Bulletin of Peace Proposals*, Vol. 20, No. 2, 1989, pp. 157–65.
Leaning, J. 'Physicians, Triage and Nuclear War', *The Lancet*. 30 July 1988, p. 269.
Leaning, J., Keyes, L. (eds.). *The Counterfeit Arc: Crisis Relocation for Nuclear War*, Bollinger Publishing Co., Massachusetts, US, 1983.
Lifton, R. J. 'On Death and Death Symbolism: The Hiroshima Disaster', *Psychiatry*, Vol. 27, 1964, pp. 191–210.
Lifton, R. J., *Death in Life*, Random House, New York, 1968.
Lifton, R. J. 'Beyond Psychic Numbing: A Call to Awareness', *American Journal of Orthopsychiatry*, Vol. 52, No. 4, 1982, pp. 619–29.
Lifton, R. J., Falk, R. *Indefensible Weapons*, Basic Books, New York, 1982.

Lowinger, P. 'The Doctor as Political Activist', *American Journal of Psychotherapy*, Vol. 22, Oct. 1968, pp. 616–25.
Lown, B. 'Physicians Confront the Nuclear Peril', *Circulation*, Vol. 72, No. 6, December 1985, pp. 1135–43.
Lown, B. *Soviet–American Cooperation: A Physician's Perspective*. IPPNW, Boston, US, 1986.
McCally, M., Cassel, C. 'Medical Responsibility and Global Environmental Change', *Annals of Internal Medicine*, Vol. 113, No. 6, 1990, pp. 467–73.
MacCurdy, J. *The Psychology of War*, Heinemann, London, 1918.
McDonald, J.W. *Further Exploration of Track Two Diplomacy*, Paper given at International Studies Association Annual Conference, London, March 1989.
Mack, A. *Peace Research in the 1980's*, Australian National University, Canberra, 1985.
Mack, J.E. 'Psychosocial Effects of the Nuclear Arms Race', *Bulletin of the Atomic Scientists*, Vol. 37, No. 4, 1981, pp. 18–23.
Mack, J.E. 'The Perception of US–Soviet Intentions and other Psychological Dimensions of the Nuclear Arms Race', *American Journal of Orthopsychiatry*, Vol. 52, No. 4, 1982, pp. 590–9.
Mack, J.E., Beardslee, W., et al. *Psychosocial aspects of nuclear developments* (Report No. 20), American Psychiatric Association, Washington DC, 1982.
Malone, D. (ed.). *Dictionary of American Biography, Vol. 3*, Charles Scribner & Sons, New York, 1935.
MAPW and MCANW. *The Medical Consequences of Nuclear War*, Spider Web, London, 1982.
Meerloo, A.M. *Total War and the Human Mind*, George Allen & Unwin Ltd., London, 1944.
Menkes, D. 'Psychological Defence Mechanisms and the Nuclear Arms Race: An Interactive Model', *Medicine and War*, Vol. 5, No. 2, 1989, pp. 80–95.
Merrington, M., Blundell, B., et al. *A List of the Papers and Correspondence of Lionel Sharples Penrose*, Publications Office, University College London, 1979.
Meurant, J. 'Inter Arma Caritas: Evolution and Nature of International Humanitarian Law', *Journal of Peace Research*, Vol. 24, No. 3, 1987, pp. 237–49.
Middleton, J. 'Health Promotion is Peace Promotion', *Health Promotion*, Vol. 2, No. 4, 1988, pp. 341–5.
Minnion, J., Bolsover P. (eds.), *The CND Story*, Allison & Busby, London, 1983.
Morawski, J., Goldstein, S. 'Psychology and Nuclear War. A Chapter in Our Legacy of Social Responsibility', *American Psychologist*, March 1985, pp. 276–84.
Nathan, O., Norden, H. *Einstein on Peace*, Shocken Books, New York, 1968.
National Council of Peace Societies. *Official Report of the Seventeenth Universal Congress of Peace, 1908*, London, 1909.
Netherlands Medical Association. *Medical Opinions on War*, Elsevier Publishing Co., Amsterdam, 1938.
Newcombe, A., Newcombe, H. *Peace Research Around The World*, Canadian Peace Research Institute, Ontario, 1969.
Nicolai, G. *The Biology of War*, J.M. Dent, London, 1919.
Nusbaumer, M., DiLorio, J. 'The Medicalisation of Nuclear Disarmament Claims', *Peace and Change*, Vol. XI, No. 1, Spring 1985, pp. 63–73.
Office of Technology Assessment. *The Effects of Nuclear War*, Croom Helm, London, 1980.
Openshaw, S. et al. *Doomsday: Britain after Nuclear Attack*, Blackwell, Oxford, 1983.

Pelican Freud Library, Vol. 12. *Civilisation, Society and Religion*, Penguin Books Ltd., England, 1985.
Penrose, L. S. *On the Objective Study of Crowd Behaviour*, H. K. Lewis & Co., London, 1952.
Penrose, M. 'Anti-war Medics Fight on', *General Practitioner*, 13 March 1981.
Penrose, M. (ed.). *The Pathogenesis of War*, Lewis, London, 1963.
Phillips, C., Ross, I. *The Nuclear Casebook – An Illustrated Guide*, Polygon Books, Edinburgh, 1983.
Polak, J. *A Short Contribution to the History of Pacifism in Poland*, published by the Organising Committee of the XXVI Universal Peace Congress, Warsaw. No date, but after 1926.
Porter, B. E. 'Leo Tolstoy', in *World Encyclopedia of Peace: Vol. 2*, Pergamon Press, Oxford, 1986, pp. 464–6.
The Preparation and Organisation of the Health Services for War. Home Defence Circular (77), DHSS, London, 1977.
Pridan, D. 'Rudolph Virchow and Social Medicine in Historical Perspective', *Medical History*, Vol. 8, No. 1, 1964, pp. 274–8.
Prinzing, F. *Epidemics Resulting from Wars*, Clarendon Press, Oxford, 1916.
Protect and Survive, HMSO, London, 1980.
Relman, A. 'Physicians, Nuclear War and Politics', *New England Journal of Medicine*, Vol. 307, No. 12, 16 Sept. 1982, pp. 744–5.
Richardson, F. *The Public and the Bomb*, Blackwood & Sons, London, 1981.
Richet, C. *L'Homme Stupide*, Paris, 1919. Trans. by Forsythe, N. and Harvey, L. *Idiot Man*, T. Werner Laurie, London, 1925.
Rivière, Joseph. *Esquisse Cliniques de Physicotherapie. (Traitement rationnel des Maladies Chroniques). Tome II*. Editions Médicales, Norbert Malone, Paris, 1932.
Rivière, Joseph. *Un Demi-Siècle de Physicotherapie. Organisation Mondiale de la Paix. Tome 111*, Imprimerie et Libraire Centrales des Chemins de Fer, Paris, 1934.
Robinson, J. 'Medicine and Peace in the Soviet Union', *Journal of MAPW*, Vol. 3, Part 2, April 1982, pp. 607–14.
Rosas, A. 'The Factors of Humanitarian Law', *Journal of Peace Research*, Vol. 24, No. 3, 1987, pp. 219–36.
Rotblat, J. *History of the Pugwash Conferences*, Taylor & Francis Ltd., London, 1962.
Rotblat, J., 'The Pugwash Conferences on Science and World Affairs', *Medicine and War*, Vol. 1, No. 1, 1985, pp. 51–4.
Roth, S. 'Civil Defence in the USA', *Medicine and War*, Vol. 1, No. 2, 1985, pp. 119–23.
Ruprecht, T., Jenssen, C. (eds.). *Askulap Oder Mars? Artze Geyen Den Kreig, Geschichte & Frieden*, Donat Verlag, Bremen, 1991.
Sandoz, Y. 'The Red Cross and Peace: Realities and Limits', *Journal of Peace Research*, Vol. 24, No. 3, 1987, pp. 287–96.
Schweitzer, A. *The Problem of Peace in the World Today. Nobel Peace Prize Address*, Adam & Charles Black, London, 1954.
Schweitzer, A. *Peace or Atomic War? (Three broadcast appeals from Oslo on April 28/29/30 1958)*, Adam & Charles Black, London, 1958.
Sepping, P. 'Civil Defence in the UK', *Medicine and War*, Vol. 1, No. 2, 1985, pp. 115–18.
Sheppard, H. R. L. *We Say 'NO'*, John Murray, London, 1935.
Sidel, V., Geiger, J., Lown, B. 'The Medical Consequences of Thermonuclear War', *New England Journal of Medicine*, Vol. 266, 1962, pp. 1126–55.
Sims, P. 'A Dilemma for Doctors', *Medicine and War*, Vol. 2, No. 3, 1986,

pp. 199–200.
Sivard, L., *World Military and Social Expenditures 1989*. World Priorities, Washington, 1989.
Study Group: Faculty of Community Medicine. 'Implications of Nuclear Weapons for Community Medicine', *Community Medicine*, Vol. 4, 1982, pp. 34–9.
Taylor, R., Young, N. (eds.). *Campaigns for Peace: British Peace Movements in the Twentieth Century*, Manchester University Press, Manchester, 1987.
Thompson, E.P. *Protest and Survive*, Russell Press Ltd., Nottingham, 1980.
Thompson, J. *Psychological Aspects of Nuclear War*, British Psychological Society and John Wiley, Chichester, 1985.
Thompson, J. 'Tribalism and the Arms Race Trap', *Medicine and War*, Vol. 4, No. 1, 1988, pp. 37–47.
Trotter, W. *Instincts of the Herd in Peace and War*, Benn, London, 1916.
Turco, R.P., Toon, O.P. *et al.* 'Nuclear Winter: Global Consequences of Multiple Nuclear Explosions', *Science*, Vol. 22, 1983, pp. 1283–92.
US Congress Joint Committee on Atomic Energy. *Biological and Environmental Effects of Nuclear War*, 1959.
Van der Linden, W.H. *The International Peace Movement, 1815–1874*, Tilleul Pubs., Amsterdam, 1987.
Vellacott, J. 'Women, Peace and Internationalism', in Chatfield, C. and van den Dungen, P. (eds.), *Peace Movements and Political Cultures*, University of Tennessee Press, Knoxville, 1988.
Verdoorn, J.A. *Mars en Aesculapius*, De Tijdstroom, Lochem, Holland, 1985.
Warner, G., Shuman, M. *Citizen Diplomats*, Continuum Press, New York, 1987.
Watkins, S. *Medicine and Labour*, Lawrence and Wishart, London, 1987.
Webber, P., Wilkinson, G., Rubin, B. *Crisis Over Cruise: A Plain Guide to the New Weapons*, Penguin Books, London, 1983.
Wiltsher, A. *Most Dangerous Women: Feminist Peace Campaigners of the Great War*, Pandora, London, 1985.
Wittner, L.S. 'The Transnational Movement against Nuclear Weapons, 1945–1986: A Preliminary Survey', in Chatfield, C. and van den Dungen, P. (eds.), *Peace Movements and Political Cultures*, University of Tennessee Press, US, 1988.
World Health Organisation. *Effects of nuclear war on health and health services: Report of the international committee of experts in medical sciences and public health*. WHO, Geneva, 1984; second edition 1987.
Young, N. 'Tradition and Innovation in the British Peace Movement: Towards an Analytical Framework', in Taylor, R. and Young, N. (eds.), *Campaigns for Peace*, Manchester University Press, UK, 1987.
Young, R. (ed.). *Why Wars Must Cease*, Macmillan, New York, 1935.
Zuelzer, W. *The Nicolai Case: A Biography*, Wayne State University Press, Detroit, 1982.
Zuelzer, W. 'Georg Friedrich Nicolai', in *World Encyclopedia of Peace: Vol. 2*, Pergamon Press, Oxford, 1986, pp. 42–5.

INDEX

Addams, Jane, 37
Air raids, 56
Alma Ata Declaration, 87, 104
American Peace Society, 21, 23
Amnesty International, Medical Group, 107
Anarchist International, 27
Angell, Norman, 35
Appeal to the Europeans (1914), 39
Appeasement, 64
Armaments spending, 32, 66, 84, 88
Arms race, 27, 45, 63, 72, 73, 78, 93, 94, 99, 105
Association médicale Internationale contre la Guerre, 30

Belgium, Medical Group for the Maintenance of Peace, 67
Benedict, Crystal, 38
Berlin Wall (1961), 73, 104
Biology of War, 40
Bismarck, 23, 24
Bolsheviks, 32, 46
British Medical Association, 55, 56, 68; political reaction to 1983 report, 83; relations with MCANW & MAPW, 82; vs. British Warfare Association, 55
Bronfenbrenner, Ury, 93

Caldicott, Helen, 78, 80
Cambridge Scientists Anti-War Group, 56
Campaign for Nuclear Disarmament, 74, 84
Capek, Karel, 57
Casualty calculations, 88
Central Board for Conscientious Objection, 62
Central Medical War Committee, 67
Chazov, Evgeny, 78

Chemical and Biological Warfare, 67, 79, 89, 90, 104
Citizen diplomacy, 88, 99
Civil Defence, 56, 73, 74, 76, 81, 85
Civil Protection, 86, 88
Civil Rights, 76
Cobden, Richard, 21
Cold War, 65, 67
Comfort, Alex, 71
Common Sense, 18
Community physicians, 85
Comprehensive Test Ban Treaty, 105
Congress of Nations, 21, 22
Conflict resolution, 96, 100, 102–3
Conservative Medical Society, 87
Conscientious objection, 36, 50, 61
Costa, Andrea, 27
Crimean War, 22
Crow, D.A., 55
Crowd behaviour, 69
Cruise missiles, 81, 86
Cuba Crisis, 73

Danish Physicians Against War, 66
Darwinism, 32, 40, 51
Death instinct, 53
de Bloch, Jean, 44
Defence mechanisms, psychological, 92, 93
Dehumanisation, 40, 94
de Ligt, Bart, 49, 59
Denial, 93
Displacement, 93
Doctor's View on War, The, 54, 90
Dodge, David Low, 20–1
Dunant, Henri, 11
Dutch Committee for the Prophylaxis of War (1930), 50

Einstein, Albert, 39, 53, 72, 91

Index

Environmental Commission of IPPNW, 105
Environmental concerns, 13, 33, 78, 79, 102
Esperanto, 33, 49
Ethical questions, 11, 67, 89

Fascism, 46
Fellowship of Reconciliation, 36
Feminism, 26, 28
First World War, 27, 28, 31, 32, 34, 35–9, 40, 42, 48, 73
Fischoff, Adolf, 23, 25–6
Franco, General, 46
Franklin, Benjamin, 17, 19
Free Trade Movement, 21, 31
Freud, Sigmund, 41, 42, 53, 69
Fried, Alfred, 24, 30, 34
Friends Medical Society, 67
Fromm, Erich, 73

Gandhi, 48, 49
General Electric, boycott of, 106
General Peace Convention (1843), 22
Geneva Conventions, 11
German Peace Union (1894), 24
Gorbachev, President, 100
Gregariousness, 41

Haddow, Alexander, 70, 72
Hague Peace Congress, 24
Hamilton, Alice, 37, 49
Herd Instinct, 41
Hitler, Adolf, 45, 54
Hodgkin, Henry, 36
Human rights, 5, 79, 80
Humanitarian Tribunal, 81
Humphrey, John, 79, 99
Hydrogen bomb, 70, 72

Idiot Man, 33
Instincts of the Herd in War and Peace, 41
Intermediate Nuclear Force Treaty, 104
International arbitration, 26, 31, 32, 37, 42
International Congress Against War and Militarism (1937), 60
International Humanitarian Law, 11
International League for Permanent Peace, 37
International mediation network, 101
International Negotiation Network, 102

International Peace Bureau, 32, 34, 35
International Physicians for the Prevention of Nuclear War, 32, 64, 66, 79, 84, 89, 92, 96, 99, 104–7
International Tribunal, 21, 31
Interparliamentary Union, 26

Jacobs, Aletta, 37, 49
Jefferson, Thomas, 18
Just War, 4, 61

Korean War, 64, 67
Kuliscioff, Anna, 26

Labour Party and MAPW, 66, 68
Ladd, William, 21
League of Nations, 31, 47, 49, 53
Letter to the Statesmen, 50
Ligue du Bien Public, 24
Logan Act, 20
Logan, George, 19–20
London Peace Congress (1908), 35
Lown, Bernard, 74, 78, 105, 107

MacCurdy, John, 43
Manifesto to the Civilised World, 39
Marx, Karl, 26
Mediation, 19, 38, 51, 96
Medical Association for the Prevention of War, 64–70, 77, 82, 97, 103
Medical Campaign Against Nuclear Weapons, 80–2
Medical curriculum, 106
Medical Foundation for the Care of Victims of Torture, 107
Medical Opinions on War, 51
Medical Peace Campaign, UK (1936), 52, 65, 69
Medical Peace research, 10
Medical prescription, 105
Medicalising peace language, 99
Mirror-imaging, 52, 93
Monnier, Henri, 35
Montessori, Maria, 58, 99
Moral concerns, 11, 56, 57
Morel, E. D., 35
Mussolini, Benito, 28, 45, 59
Mutual Assured Destruction, 77

Nansen, Fridjof, 49
National Peace Council, 35
Nazi Party, 13, 38, 46

Netherlands Association for Medical Polemology (NVMP), 77
New Left, 77
Nicolai, Georg Friedrich, 39, 69, 98
Nilsson, Nils, 34
No Conscription Fellowship, 35
No More War Movement, 49
Nobel Peace Prize, 32, 60, 71, 74, 80
Non-government organisations, 101–3, 106
Nuclear testing, 73, 75, 78, 105
Nuclear war, 67, 75
Nuclear Weapons Free Zone, 72
Nuclear winter, 88

Oaths, Hippocratic, 15, 67, 87, 91; Declaration of Geneva, 15

Paine, Thomas, 18
Partial Test Ban Treaty, 75
Peace concepts, 3, 4
Peace Conferences (1818–51), 24
Peace Congress, 22
Peace education, 9, 31
Peace Movements, 1; goals and objectives, 5; peaks and troughs, 6; traditions, 7, 98
Peace Pledge Union, 48, 57
Peace research, 8
Peace Society, First, 20
Peace Studies, 8
Peace Through Strength, 6
Pelletier, Madeleine, 26, 28–9
Penrose, Lionel, 69, 103
Pershing missiles, 81
Physicians for Social Responsibility, 74, 78
Physicotherapy, 31
Polak, J., 34
Polish Peace Society, 34
Potonie-Pierre, Edmond, 24
Primitive Instinct, 42
Proliferation, of nuclear weapons, 81, 104
Protect and Survive, 81, 86
Protest and Survive, 86
Psychiatry, contributions to peace, 91
Psychic numbing, 77, 94
Psychologists for Peace, 53
Psychology, contributions to peace, 91
PUGWASH, 72

Quakers, 19, 21, 36, 69

Red Cross, 11, 29, 49, 60, 66

Responsibilities, social, political and ethical, 12
Richet, Charles, 12, 32–3, 40, 66
Richet, Charles (Jnr), 66
Rivière, Joseph, 30–2, 35, 99
Role-models, 1, 98
Royal Army Medical Corps, 58
Rush, Benjamin, 16–19
Russell, Bertrand, 35, 72, 74
Russian Revolution (1917), 46
Russo-Japanese War, 30
Ryle, John, 54, 57

SANE, 73
SatelLife, 105
Schauta, F., 34
Schweitzer, Albert, 71, 73
Scientists Against Nuclear Arms, 88
Scientists for Peace, 68
Second World War, 38, 46, 54, 58, 61
Sheppard, Dick, 57, 61
Skarvan, Albert, 12, 29
Slavery, 18, 22, 26
Social responsibilities, 11
Socialist influences, 26–9, 46
Spanish Civil War, 46, 48
Spock, Benjamin, 73
Sputnik, 73
Stereotyping, 93
Suttner, Bertha, 34
Swedish Peace Union/League, 34
Swiss Peace Society, 35

Three Mile Island, 78
Tolstoy, Leo, 29
Torture, 15, 90, 107
Track Two Diplomacy, 100–1, 103
Triage, 89, 90
Tribal Instinct, 39, 41
Trident submarines, 81
Triple Crisis (1936), 48, 52
Trotter, Wilfred, 41, 43, 69
Turati, Filippo, 27

Union of Democratic Control, 35
United Nations, 70, 102
United Nations Second Assembly, 103
United Peace Fellowship, 35
Universal Peace Congress, 31, 32

Vienna Peace Congress (1952), 69

Index

Vietnam War, 13, 39, 63, 72, 76
Virchow, Rudolph, 12, 23–25, 98

War Resisters International, 49
War toys, 51
White Sickness, The, 57
Women's International League for Peace and Freedom, 7, 49

Women's suffrage, 28, 29, 37
World Disarmament Campaign, 82
World Health Organisation, 85, 87
World Peace Council, 64, 69

Yellow fever, 18

Zamenhof, L., 33